Clinical Investigation of Skin Disorders

JOIN US ON THE INTERNET VIA WWW, GOPHER, FTP OR EMAIL:

WWW: http://www.thomson.com
GOPHER: gopher.thompson.com
FTP: ftp.thompson.com
EMAIL: findit@kiosk.thompson.com

A service of I(T)P®

Clinical Investigation of Skin Disorders

Edited by

Rino Cerio BSc, MB BS (Lond), FRCP Edin, FRCP DipRCPath
Consultant Dermatologist and Senior Lecturer in Dermatopathology
The Royal London and St Bartholomew's Hospitals
(University of London)
London, UK

Clive B. Archer BSc, MB BS, MD, PhD (Lond), FRCP Edin, FRCP
Consultant Dermatologist and Clinical Senior Lecturer in Medicine
University of Bristol
Bristol Royal Infirmary (UBHT)
Bristol, UK

CHAPMAN & HALL MEDICAL
London · Weinheim · New York · Tokyo · Melbourne · Madras

Published by

Chapman & Hall, an imprint of Thomson Science, 2—6 Boundary Row, London SE1 8HN, UK

Thomson Science, 2—6 Boundary Row, London˙ SE1 8HN, UK

Thomson Science, 115 Fifth Avenue, New York, NY 10003, USA

Thomson Science, Suite 750, 400 Market Street, Philadelphia, PA 19106, USA

Thomson Science, Pappelallee 3, 69469 Weinheim, Germany

First edition 1998

c 1998 Chapman & Hall

Thomson Science is a division of International Thomson Publishing

Printed in Spain by
Artes Gráficas Toledo, S.A.
D.L. TO: 1865-1997
ISBN   0 412 59230 4

A catalogue record for this book is available from the British Library

Contents

Contributors

Clive B. Archer BSc, MB BS, MD, PhD (Lond),
  FRCP Edin, FRCP
Consultant Dermatologist and
  Clinical Senior Lecturer in Medicine
University of Bristol
Bristol Royal Infirmary (UBHT)
Bristol, UK

Rino Cerio BSc, MB BS, FRCP Edin, FRCP
  DipRCPath
Consultant Dermatologist and Senior Lecturer in
  Dermatopathology
The Royal London and St Bartholomew's Hospitals
  (University of London)
London, UK

Rodney P. R. Dawber MA, MB ChB, FRCP
Consultant Dermatologist
Churchill Hospital
Oxford, UK

David A.R. de Berker BA, MB BS, MRCP (UK)
Consultant Dermatologist and Honorary Clinical
  Senior Lecturer
University of Bristol
Bristol Royal Infirmary (UBHT)
Bristol, UK

M. Giles S. Dunnill MB BS, MD, MRCP (UK)
Consultant Dermatologist and Honorary Clinical
  Senior Lecturer
University of Bristol
Bristol Royal Infirmary (UBHT)
Bristol, UK

Robin A.J. Eady MB BS, FRCP
Professor of Dermatology
St John's Institute of Dermatology
St Thomas' Hospital
London, UK

Dee Anna Glaser MD
Senior Resident in Dermatology
Saint Louis University School of Medicine
Division of Dermatology
St Louis, USA

Elizabeth M. Johnson BSc, PhD
Clinical Scientist
PHLS Mycology Reference Laboratory
Public Health Laboratory
Bristol, UK

John P. Leeming BSc, PhD
Clinical Scientist
Public Health Laboratory
Bristol Royal Infirmary
Bristol, UK

Christopher R. Lovell MB ChB, MD (Bristol),
  FRCP
Consultant Dermatologist
Royal United Hospital
Bath, UK

Gillian M. Murphy MB BCh BAO, MD (Cork)
  FRCPI
Consultant Dermatologist
Beaumont and Mater Misericordiae Hospitals
Dublin, Ireland

Neal S. Penneys MD, PhD
Professor and Chairman of Dermatology and
  Dermatopathology
Saint Louis University School of Medicine
Division of Dermatology
St Louis, USA

Jane C. Sterling MA, MB BChir, PhD, MRCP (UK)
Honorary Consultant Dermatologist and MRC
  Clinical Scientist Fellow
Addenbrooke's Hospital
Cambridge, UK

David W. Warnock BSc, PhD, MRCPath
Consultant Clinical Scientist in Mycology
PHLS Mycology Reference Laboratory
Public Health Laboratory
Bristol, UK

Preface

Doctors (and patients) are often surprised to discover that there are nearly 2000 different skin disorders – a fact which, no doubt, contributes to the mystery of dermatology for many physicians. Depending on variations in medical practice worldwide, common and uncommon skin disorders may present to a wide range of clinicians, including specialist dermatologists, family practitioners and hospital doctors.

The aim of this book is to acquaint the physician with an up-to-date systematic approach to the investigation of patients with medical and surgical disorders of the skin. By concentrating on clinical investigation, important information is made readily available to the reader, thereby avoiding the need to search painstakingly through larger general dermatology tomes.

Emphasizing the need for the skilled clinical assessment of the dermatology patient, subsequent chapters are arranged to provide a logical and practical approach to clinical investigation. In recognition of the importance of visual stimuli to the learning process, we have made efforts to include many clinical photographs and illustrations.

Chapter 1 describes how to take a dermatological history in the context of the general medical setting, before carrying out the clinical examination and, if indicated, simple bedside investigations. We have included several practical tips such as how to guess the diagnosis from the referral letter and the good sense of taking an early glimpse at the problem to help direct the clinical history. Chapter 2 on dermatopathology covers how and when to do a skin biopsy, when to avoid a skin biopsy, common examples of histopathological patterns and how to interpret a histopathology report. There follow chapters on general laboratory investigations, investigation of allergic skin disorders and the photodermatoses, bacteriology and mycology, tests for viral, HIV-related and tropical infections, and investigation of hair and nail disorders. Looking to the future, we have also included chapters on prenatal diagnosis of heritable skin diseases and the application of molecular biology techniques in dermatology.

The editing of this book has been fairly rigorous in order to provide a uniform style of presentation, and we are most grateful to our co-contributors for their input and tolerance. We are also grateful to contributors for providing photographs for individual chapters and, in particular, to Stuart Robertson of the Department of Medical Illustration at the St John's Institute of Dermatology, London.

This book provides a rational overview of the clinical investigation of the majority of skin disorders. It is written in a lively manner and should be of great value to dermatologists, dermatology residents, family practitioners and other specialist physicians.

Rino Cerio and Clive B. Archer

Chapter 1

Clinical assessment of the dermatology patient

Clive B. Archer

1

Dermatology is historically a general medical specialty but in recent years there has been an increasing emphasis on the surgical aspects of managing skin disorders. This trend is partly due to the success of skin cancer public information programmes. 'It is patently clear that proper management of the patient, whether medical or surgical, can only be planned once the correct diagnosis has been made'. This is an admirable sentiment which applies to the whole of medicine. If only it were true! Any experienced clinician will be able to think of examples where the patient was managed correctly despite an incorrect diagnosis. Nevertheless, as clinicians we should strive to practice medicine, be it an art or a science (or perhaps an art based on science), to the best of our ability and this means aiming to make the right diagnosis most of the time.

Since the number of different skin diseases has been estimated at nearly 2000, one should not expect to develop instant expertise. It is possible to manage a patient appropriately without detailed knowledge of all the benign adnexal tumours but the old adage that there are only two dermatoses: those that are steroid-responsive and those that are not, displays an outdated lack of knowledge that not even professors can get away with. A reasonable knowledge of dermatology is essential for all doctors who look after patients. Skin diseases are common, accounting for about 15% of family practitioner consultations.

A logical approach to the clinical assessment of the dermatology patient will provide a sound basis upon which to build. Once a clinical diagnosis or differential diagnosis has been made, one can then plan the management of the patient. This will include decisions about appropriate clinical investigations (as discussed in subsequent chapters) and good clinical assessment may well save the patient expensive and unnecessary investigations.

As in other aspects of medicine, the diagnosis of skin disorders depends on taking a detailed but well-directed history followed by examination of the patient and sometimes the performance of simple bedside tests and/or further clinical investigations. In order to maintain one's interest amidst busy clinics, it can be fun to guess the diagnosis from the referral letter but this activity should never replace the sound clinical skills of history-taking and clinical examination. There is usually no time for an exhaustive general medical history and in many instances this would be inappropriate. However, one should avoid considering the dermatological problem in isolation from the patient's general medical setting and social circumstances. The consultation should allow sufficient time not only to make the correct diagnosis but also to explain to the patient, in terms that can be understood, the natural history and management of the particular skin disorder.

With experience, the referral letter or an early glimpse of the skin disorder can allow one to focus the history and, in some cases, the history will allow fine tuning of the diagnosis. For example, a detailed personal, family and social history will help the clinician decide whether a patient with hand eczema has exogenous or endogenous hand eczema, possibly a manifestation of atopic dermatitis (atopic eczema). An important function of taking a history is to allow the establishment of a rapport between the doctor and patient before the clinical examination is performed.

It is debatable whether one should elicit first a general history or dermatological history from the patient. I find it more rewarding to concentrate on the presenting complaint and to follow this by an expanded dermatological history before taking a directed general history.

DERMATOLOGICAL HISTORY

Having established the age, sex and racial origin of the patient and sometimes being led by the referral letter, I usually ask the patient to: **'Describe in your own words what has been troubling you with your skin and when it started'.**

Patients vary in their ability to tell a concise, relevant story and the need for the doctor to interrupt tactfully will depend on this ability. It is usually possible to establish quickly whether one is dealing with a rash (such as eczema or psoriasis) or a skin lesion or lesions.

Dermatologists do not favour use of the term skin rash and will offer cogent arguments based on the fact that, to their knowledge, rashes do not affect other organs of the body. One should try to avoid asking leading questions, but we all do it. Patients sometimes use words incorrectly. For example, a patient with urticaria may describe a wheal as a blister and close questioning is required to establish that the patient has not actually seen any fluid-filled cavities.

Helpful prompts include:

- **How did it start?**
- **What did it look like?**
- **How did it develop?**
- **When exactly did it begin?**
- **Have you had this before?**
- **Did anything make it worse or better?**

For example, did the rash begin in the summer and only occur on sunny days? Could the rash be related to the ingestion of a food or a recently prescribed drug? A list of concurrent medications and when each was started should help answer this question.

One should ask about previous treatments, especially topical treatments, either prescribed or purchased as over-the-counter preparations. Some of these treatments may have helped whereas others may have made matters worse. For example, a potent fluorinated topical corticosteroid is sometimes erroneously applied to the face, leading to a perioral dermatitis; a fungal infection of the skin may worsen after the application of a topical corticosteroid, producing tinea incognita; the patient may have become allergic to a local anaesthetic or preservative in a topical preparation used to alleviate pruritus ani.

It can be useful to ask early on: **'Was the rash itchy?'** and **'Did the skin become dry, scaly, flaky, crusted or weepy?'** Itching in the absence of epidermal changes is often due to urticaria (Fig. 1.1) and the history of intermittent whealing, of variable duration, sometimes associated with subcutaneous swelling (angioedema) may become evident. Severely itchy, excoriated, crusted skin may be due to a form of eczema or the mite infestation, scabies. Any suspicion of scabies should lead to the question: **'Are any other family members or friends itching?'**

Generalized pruritus, in the absence of any rash or skin lesions, would lead one to consider general medical causes of itching (Chapter 3).

If it becomes apparent that the presenting complaint is a skin lesion, either a benign or malignant skin tumour, the history is often directed by the clinical impression gained from an early glimpse of the lesion. The history of a slowly enlarging lesion developing over a few months on a sun-exposed site would be consistent with a basal cell epithelioma (basal cell carcinoma) or squamous cell carcinoma, whereas a rapidly growing lesion developing over a period of a few weeks would be more consistent with a keratoacanthoma (Fig. 1.2). A rapid diagnosis of viral warts or molluscum contagiosum warts may render a detailed history unnecessary but, particularly in an adult, one might need to consider the possibility of immunosuppression and question the patient appropriately.

With increased awareness of the dangers of excessive sun exposure, patients are often concerned about the possibility of a benign melanocytic naevus or naevi changing into a malignant melanoma (Fig. 1.3). Specific questions may include:

- **How long have you had this mole?**
- **In what way has it changed? Over what period of time?**

Fig. 1.1 Urticaria, showing red raised itchy transient wheals on the back.

- **Has it become larger?**
- **Has it changed shape or colour?**
- **Has it bled or become itchy?**

Spontaneous bleeding of a melanocytic lesion is more worrying than bleeding as a result of minor injury. In my experience, itching alone is usually not a sign of malignant change but this symptom would take on more significance in the presence of other changes. Again, one should try to avoid leading the patient too much in a particular direction and, in this instance, the clinical appearance

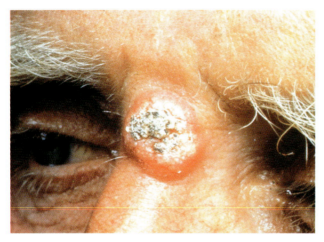

Fig. 1.2 Keratoacanthoma, showing a solitary dome-shaped lesion on the bridge of the nose.

of the pigmented lesion or lesions will be particularly important. For example, these changing features would be perfectly acceptable in a seborrhoeic keratosis, which may be one of multiple lesions as one sees with benign melanocytic naevi (Fig. 1.4).

GENERAL HISTORY

With experience the general history will become well-directed as a result of information gained from the dermatological history. If necessary, one should ask further questions related to past medical history, family history and social history including occupation, leisure activities, home situation and travel overseas. One should also form an opinion about the patient's psychological state, although stress should not be blamed too readily as the cause of the skin disease.

Past medical history

An exhaustive history of past medical illnesses is not always required and this aspect of the consultation should be directed, to an extent, by the presenting complaint. A previous history of skin diseases such as psoriasis or eczema may be relevant or incidental to the present problem. If early impressions point to a form of eczema, perhaps

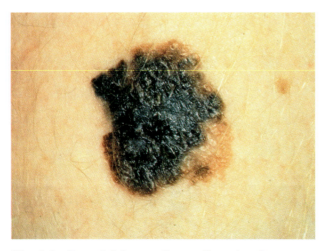

Fig. 1.3 Superficial spreading malignant melanoma, in which a long-standing naevus on the trunk rapidly became darker in colour.

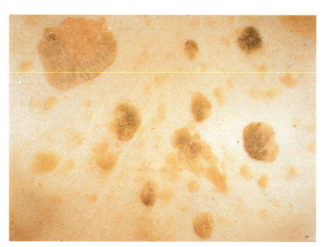

Fig. 1.4 Seborrhoeic keratoses, showing numerous light brown rough-surfaced lesions on the trunk.

atopic dermatitis, one should ask specifically about childhood eczema, asthma or hay fever. A patient with alopecia areata may also have vitiligo or other autoimmune diseases, including thyroiditis, diabetes mellitus and pernicious anaemia.

Enquiry about past medical illnesses should include a history of prescribed drugs and over-the-counter medications. A general medical disease may be directly relevant to the dermatological disorder. For example, long-standing arthritis may prove to be psoriatic rather than another seronegative arthritis after all, and gastric symptoms may underlie iron-deficiency anaemia with resultant diffuse hair loss.

Family history

Questions related to family history frequently follow on from the past medical history. There may well be a family history of psoriasis, atopic disorders or autoimmune diseases. It is important to take care in the interpretation of this aspect of the patient's history, however. The apparent occurrence of allergies within the family can be particularly misleading.

A patient with an inherited disease such as neurofibromatosis may not volunteer a family history. Not all familial diseases are genetic in origin and a family history of pruritus in a patient with scabies may only become apparent on direct questioning.

Social history

The social history should include details of occupation, leisure activities, the home situation and travel abroad.

When the occupation seems to be relevant to the skin disorder, as may be the case in hand eczema, one should find out precisely what the patient does at work. What materials are handled? Is protective clothing and/or gloves worn? What are the gloves made of? Sometimes a work-related skin disorder will settle down when the patient is absent from work, either on sick leave or on holiday. This is not always true,

however: the chronic hand eczema of chromate sensitivity in cement workers is well-known to persist after the allergen has been removed from the patient or vice versa.

Individuals with a background of atopic dermatitis or other manifestations of atopy, however mild, can develop severe, persistent hand eczema as hairdressers, caterers or nurses. This emphasizes the need for good career advice during the teenage years.

Leisure activities are an important aspect of most people's lives. Sporting activities may be associated with exacerbations of skin disorders. For example, sweating may irritate the skin of patients with atopic dermatitis, exercise can induce cholinergic urticaria, and impetigo can run riot in a rugby scrum! Hobbies such as photography can lead to the handling of irritant or sensitizing chemicals. One should enquire about personal habits, including the application of cosmetics (that is, make-up, perfume, nail varnish, aftershave), the wearing of costume jewellery and the colouring of hair.

A dusty home environment can cause exacerbations of atopic dermatitis, as can cigarette smoke. The home situation can be an important factor in the management of patients with skin disorders. Some patients will be unable to treat their skin adequately at home, either through lack of amenities, such as a bath, or because of a busy or disorganized lifestyle.

A knowledge of recent travel abroad, even for a short time, may be crucial to making the correct diagnosis. For example, it is not uncommon to see the occasional traveller with leishmaniasis or a tourist with cutaneous larva migrans (creeping eruption).

EXAMINING THE DERMATOLOGY PATIENT

Physical examination of the patient is an important part of making the correct diagnosis. One should always consider the patient as a whole and avoid merely focusing on the skin or a minute aspect of it. A magnifying glass can be a useful tool but a view of the doctor's face through the magnifying glass as he or she enters the room is probably no great comfort to the patient.

The examination should take place in a room with a good source of light, preferably daylight. A lesion of uncertain diagnosis when viewed in a dim light can become in a good light an obvious basal cell epithelioma, with pearly appearance and traversing telangiectasia. In most cases the whole of the skin (or at least the vast majority of it) should be examined, with the patient wearing underclothes only. **Window dermatology** (an original term, Archer 1995), in which limited areas of the skin are offered and examined, is not good clinical practice and could be dangerous practice with consequent medicolegal implications. A good dermatologist will always consider the possibility of a concealed malignant melanoma and, for this reason along with the wish to provide a proper medical service to patients, will be reluctant to offer a dermatological opinion in the hospital corridor to even the most esteemed of medical colleagues.

The hair and nails are important skin appendages and the oral mucosa should be examined in many instances, if not routinely; the genital mucosal surfaces should be examined if indicated. Lichen planus (Fig. 1.5) is an example of a skin disease which commonly affects the buccal mucosa (sometimes other mucosal surfaces) and may be associated with nail dystrophy and scarring alopecia.

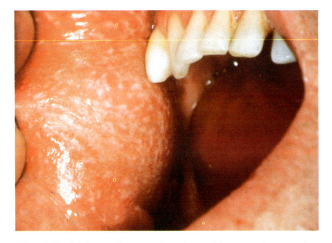

Fig. 1.5 Lichen planus, showing white papules on the buccal mucosa.

When examining the skin, it is usual to consider the form or morphology of individual lesions, the overall distribution on the body, and the pattern of the lesions in relation to each other. In practice (and with experience) these three assessments are made almost simultaneously and many skin disorders become instantly recognizable.

Morphology

A list of commonly used dermatology terms is shown in Table 1.1. Lesions may be solitary or multiple. A rash (or eruption) describes the complete picture of multiple lesions and its use should not be restricted to a description of a confluent red rash, as seen, for example, in measles. A maculopapular rash, strangely enough, consists of both macules and papules.

It is usual to describe the size, colour, consistency (is it soft or firm?), shape, margins (is there a sharp or diffuse edge?) and surface characteristics of skin lesions. For example, one might refer to a large brown rough-surfaced seborrhoeic keratosis, a small firm reddish dermatofibroma or a large soft lipoma with diffuse edge.

The shape of the lesions can point to the diagnosis and it is often useful to consider which level of the skin is involved (for example, is this an epidermal or dermal problem?; Fig. 1.6). Table 1.2 shows a simplified classification of skin diseases according to the predominant level of pathology in the skin, although in some disorders more than one level will be involved.

Annular lesions or plaques are commonly seen. Epidermal changes, such as scaling, crusting, excoriation and lichenification, occur in psoriasis, discoid eczema (Fig. 1.7), tinea corporis (ringworm; Fig. 1.8), pityriasis rosea, lichen planus and secondary syphilis. Granulomatous change in the dermis, giving rise to a slightly knobbly appearance of the skin, is seen in granuloma annulare, sarcoidosis, lupus vulgaris (a form of cutaneous tuberculosis) and leprosy. Erythema or oedema in the dermal layer is more likely to represent urticaria, erythema multiforme or an annular erythema.

Table 1.1 Dermatological terminology

Lesion	Any single small area of skin pathology
Macule	An area of colour change
Papule	A small* elevated (palpable) lesion
Wheal	An oedematous slightly raised lesion, often with a pale centre and reddish margin
Nodule	A large* elevated spherical lesion, often extending deeply into the skin
Plaque	A flat-topped palpable lesion
Vesicle	A small fluid-filled blister
Pustule	A small blister filled with neutrophils (pus)
Bulla	A large fluid-filled blister
Purpura	A visible collection of free red blood cells in the skin
Scale	Thickened fragments of the outermost layer of the epidermis, the statum corneum
Crust	Dried plasma exudate
Excoriation	An abrasion caused by scratching
Lichenification	Area of increased epidermal thickness and increased skin markings as a result of chronic rubbing
Erosion	An absence of the epithelial surface
Ulcer	An absence of the epithelial surface with dermal damage (i.e. deeper than an erosion)
Scar	A permanent lesion resulting from repair by replacement with connective tissue
Telangiectasia	Dilated blood vessels visible on the skin surface

* It is not usually helpful to be dogmatic about precise measurements.

Table 1.2 Dermatoses according to the level of pathology within the skin

Predominant change/site of pathology	Disease
Epidermal changes (e.g. scaling, hyperkeratosis, crusting)	Psoriasis, eczema/dermatitis, superficial fungal infections, the ichthyoses
Epidermal appendages	Acne vulgaris, rosacea, hidradenitis suppurativa (apocrine glands in axillae and groin), alopecia areata
Dermo–epidermal interface and dermis	Pityriasis rosea, lichen planus, lupus erythematosus, erythema multiforme
Epidermal and dermo–epidermal cohesion (blistering disorders)	Pemphigus (e.g. vulgaris/foliaceus), pemphigoid, dermatitis herpetiformis, epidermolysis bullosa
Dermis	The urticarias, granuloma annulare, morphoea/scleroderma, dermatomyositis, xanthoma/xanthelasma, lymphoma (e.g. T-cell lymphoma/mycosis fungoides)
Subcutaneous tissue	Erythema nodosum and other forms of panniculitis

Fig. 1.6   Diagrammatic view of the skin.

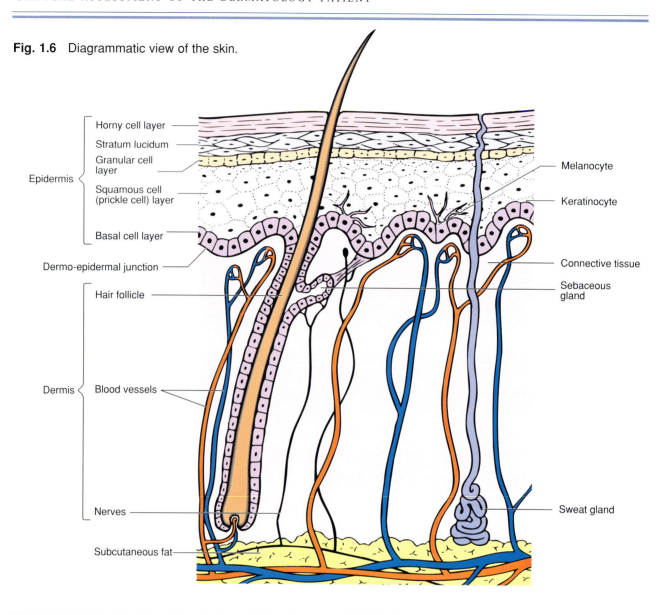

Fig. 1.7   Discoid (nummular) eczema, showing itchy circular crusted plaques on the arm.

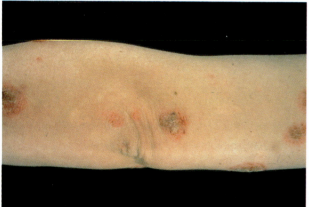

Fig. 1.8   Tinea corporis, showing red scaly circular plaques on the thigh; central clearing and an advancing inflamed border are characteristic.

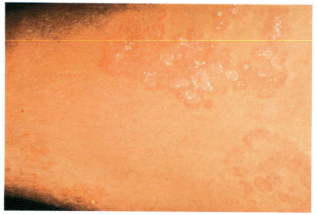

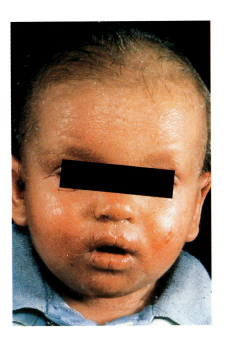

Fig. 1.9 Atopic dermatitis in infancy, showing typical involvement of the face.

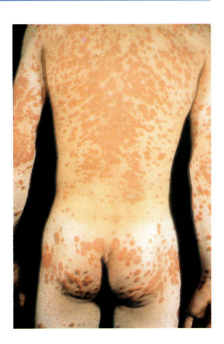

Fig. 1.10 Psoriasis, showing erythematous inflammatory plaques on the trunk, elbows and buttocks.

Table 1.3 A classification of the eczemas	
Endogenous	*Exogenous*
Atopic dermatitis	Irritant dermatitis
Discoid eczema	Allergic contact dermatitis
Asteatotic eczema	Seborrhoeic dermatitis*
Pompholyx	Photodermatitis
Varicose (venous) eczema	Drug-induced eczema

*Predominantly due to Pityrosporon yeasts

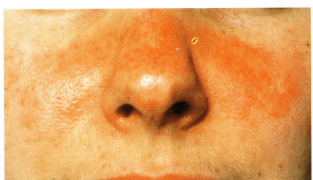

Fig. 1.11 Seborrhoeic dermatitis, showing redness and scaling of the nose and paranasal regions. Rosacea frequently accompanies seborrhoeic eczema.

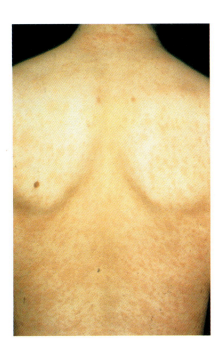

Fig. 1.12 Pityriasis rosea, showing the typical 'Christmas tree' distribution of oval, sometimes slightly scaly, macules on the trunk.

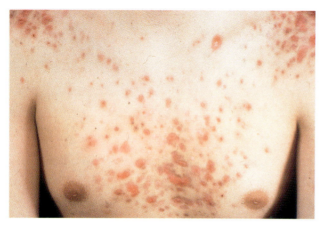

Fig. 1.13 Acne vulgaris, showing scarring nodulo-cystic lesions on the chest and shoulders.

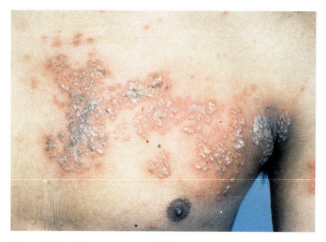

Fig. 1.15 Herpes zoster (shingles), showing inflammatory blisters and crusts on the left side of the chest.

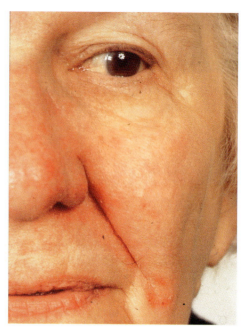

Fig. 1.14 Rosacea, showing erythema, telangiectasia and papules on the cheek.

Distribution

Skin lesions may be localized or widespread. Although there will be many exceptions, several characteristic distributions exist and common skin disorders are often symmetrical. A unilateral scaly annular rash may be due to a fungal infection.

In children and adults, atopic dermatitis tends to affect the antecubital and popliteal fossae, the periocular regions and nape of the neck as well as other areas if severe. In infancy, atopic dermatitis affects the face and extensor aspects of the limbs (Fig. 1.9) whereas flexural eczema at this age, with scalp involvement, is characteristic of seborrhoeic eczema (seborrhoeic dermatitis). The terms

eczema and dermatitis are best used synonymously and there are several types (Table 1.3).

Psoriasis characteristically involves the elbows, knees, extensor aspects of the limbs and the scalp, particularly the scalp margins (Fig. 1.10). Seborrhoeic dermatitis in adults usually affects the scalp, paranasal regions, eyebrows and sometimes the presternal area, the interscapular skin and flexures (Fig. 1.11). Pityriasis rosea presents with red scaly, oval plaques on the chest and back. There is usually a characteristic 'Christmas tree' arrangement of the lesions on the back and, with the exception of the upper thighs, the legs are largely spared (Fig. 1.12).

Acne vulgaris occurs on the face, chest and back (Fig. 1.13), reflecting the distribution of the sebaceous glands, whereas acne rosacea (in which comedones are absent) is nearly always confined to the face (Fig. 1.14), being a more common cause of a facial eruption of 'butterfly' distribution than the much quoted rash of systemic lupus erythematosus.

In addition to the shape of individual lesions and their distribution, the **pattern** in which

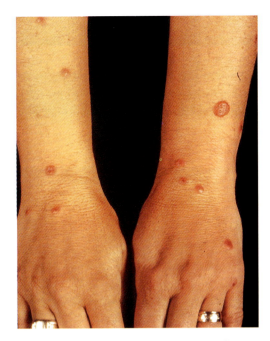

Fig. 1.16 Insect bites, showing persistent inflammatory lesions on the forearms.

Table 1.4 Skin disorders according to body regions	
Region	*Skin disorder*
Face	Acne vulgaris
	Rosacea
	Facial eczema
	Seborrhoeic dermatitis
	Contact dermatitis
	(Atopic dermatitis)
	Lupus erythematosus
	(Psoriasis)
Trunk	Acne vulgaris
	Psoriasis
	Pityriasis rosea
	Pityriasis/tinea versicolor
	(Seborrhoeic dermatitis)
	Drug eruption
Limbs	Atopic dermatitis
	Psoriasis
	Discoid eczema
	Lichen planus
	(Varicose/venous eczema)
Hands and feet	Pompholyx
	Contact dermatitis
	Atopic dermatitis
	Psoriasis
	Tinea
	Scabies
Flexures	Tinea
	Psoriasis
	Seborrhoeic dermatitis
	Hidradenitis suppurativa
	Erythrasma
Scalp	Psoriasis
	Seborrhoeic dermatitis
	Tinea capitis
	Lupus erythematosus
	Lichen planus

lesions are arranged may be characteristic. The two main patterns are linear and grouped lesions.

Linear lesions may be of developmental origin, as one sees with epidermal naevi, or determined by the Köbner or isomorphic phenomenon, in which skin lesions are localized to a site of injury such as scratch or scar. This can occur in psoriasis, lichen planus, plane warts or molluscum contagiosum warts. Herpes zoster (shingles) follows the distribution of a peripheral nerve; pain or tenderness frequently precedes the characteristic vesicular eruption (Fig. 1.15). Contact with exogenous materials is often linear, the linear blisters and streaky pigmentation of a phytophotodermatitis being a striking example. Grouped papules or nodules, particularly on the lower legs, should alert the physician to the possibility of insect bites (Fig. 1.16).

Having emphasized the need to look at the patient as a whole, it can be useful to think of a differential diagnosis based on the region or regions of the body involved (Table 1.4).

A good **clinical photography** service is desirable and in some situations, the examination of previous photographs of lesions is an essential part of managing the patient (for example, when looking for changes in a patient with multiple atypical naevi). There will be occasions when a general medical examination will be required and there is often the need to look for signs of anaemia, altered thyroid function (as in diffuse hair loss), lymphadenopathy or hepatomegaly (for example, in assessment of a patient with a skin tumour or lymphoma).

Recognizing skin disorders in black skin

Redness of the skin can be helpful in identifying skin diseases such as psoriasis or atopic dermatitis but this sign may be difficult to assess in deeply pigmented or black skin. Post-inflammatory hyperpigmentation or post-inflammatory hypopigmentation may form the predominant colour changes.

In inflammatory disorders such as atopic dermatitis, acne vulgaris and lichen planus, the post-inflammatory hyperpigmentation can persist well after the active disease process has subsided and sometimes indefinitely. Post-inflammatory hyperpigmentation particularly occurs in diseases which affect the basal layer of the epidermis, such as lichen planus or lupus erythematosus (Fig.

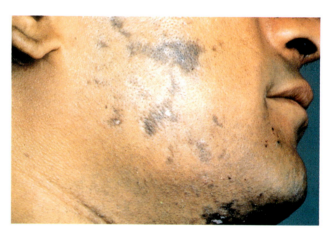

Fig. 1.17 Discoid lupus erythematosus, showing post-inflammatory hyperpigmentation on the face of a man with deeply pigmented skin.

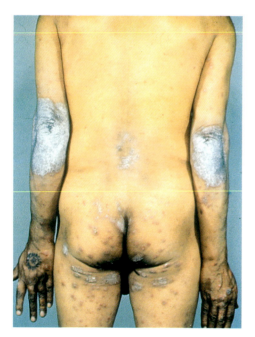

Fig. 1.18 Psoriasis, showing grey hyperkeratotic plaques on the elbows, trunk, buttocks and thighs.

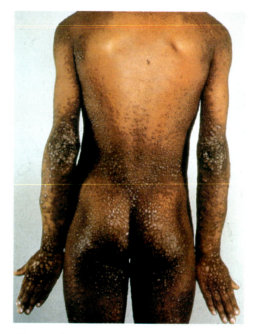

Fig. 1.19 Atopic dermatitis in black skin, showing thick lichenified lesions, particularly over the elbows and extensor surfaces (the so-called reverse pattern).

1.17), when melanin spills into the upper dermis to be engulfed by macrophages (pigmentary incontinence). Post-inflammatory hypopigmentation may occur in psoriasis and atopic dermatitis and hyper- and hypopigmentation are sometimes seen together. Black patients sometimes use over-the-counter bleaching creams, containing hydroquinone, which can paradoxically lead to an increase in skin pigmentation, termed exogenous or acquired ochronosis.

In black skin, papulosquamous diseases, such as psoriasis, frequently have a violaceous colour, with overlying grey scale, and the distribution of the eruption is an important factor in making a diagnosis (Fig. 1.18). The distribution of the lesions may be different from the characteristic pattern in white skin, as seen with atopic dermatitis, in which the elbows, knees and extensor aspects of the limbs can be involved in the so-called reverse pattern (Fig. 1.19). The lesions can also be accentuated around hair follicles (follicular eczema). The shape and pattern of individual lesions and consideration of which level of skin is involved will be essential for the diagnosis of disorders such as sarcoidosis (more common in black skin; Fig. 1.20) or an annular erythema, in which no erythema may be seen.

In addition to cutaneous sarcoidosis, other skin diseases, including keloids and pseudofolliculitis barbae, occur more frequently in black skin. Keloids (Fig. 1.21), either induced by trauma or spontaneous, can be devastating to the patient and very difficult to treat. In pseudofolliculitis barbae (Fig. 1.22), the shaved curved hairs penetrate the skin to set up a foreign-body reaction resulting in papules, pustules and sometimes prominent post-inflammatory hyperpigmentation. One should consider the possibility of diseases such as leprosy in patients who have lived in tropical countries.

Normal variants in black skin include palmar pits in the skin creases, which themselves are sometimes darkly pigmented, asymptomatic pigmentation on the oral mucosa, nail pigmenta-

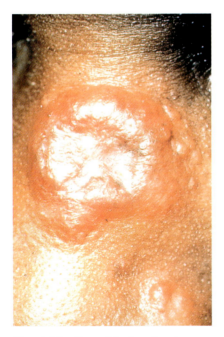

Fig. 1.20 Sarcoidosis, showing dermal annular lesions on the nose in a man of Afro-Caribbean origin.

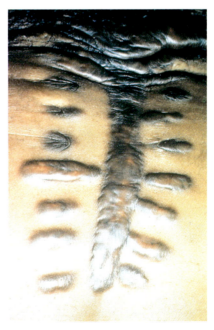

Fig. 1.21 Keloids in black skin, following an abdominal operation.

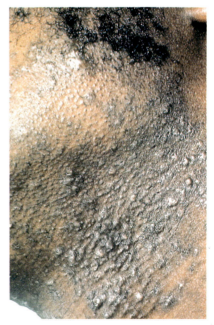

Fig. 1.22 Pseudofolliculitis barbae, affecting the face and neck. This is relatively common in black men.

tion, hyperpigmented macules on the soles of the feet and Futcher's or Voigt's line of demarcation between dark and light skin on the upper arms.

CLINICAL INVESTIGATIONS

The clinical investigation of skin disorders will depend, to an extent, on the diagnostic acumen of the physician who should aim to carry out well-directed relevant tests, thereby avoiding expensive and unnecessary investigations.

As discussed in subsequent chapters, dermatological investigations may include the need for histopathological examination of the skin; general laboratory investigations; allergy and photobiology tests; mycology and bacteriology investigations; tests for viral, HIV-related and tropical skin infections; and hair and nail investigations.

Fig. 1.23 (a, b) Wood's light demonstration of tinea capitis, showing blue fluorescence.

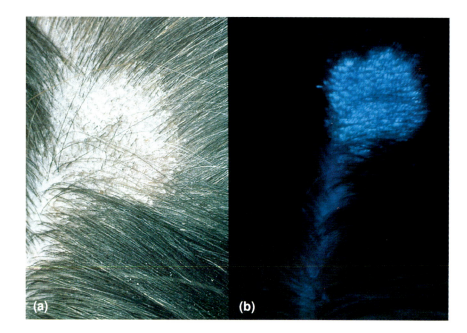

Fig. 1.24 (a, b) Erythrasma, showing a hyper-pigmented plaque in the right axilla, with coral-red fluorescence under Wood's light.

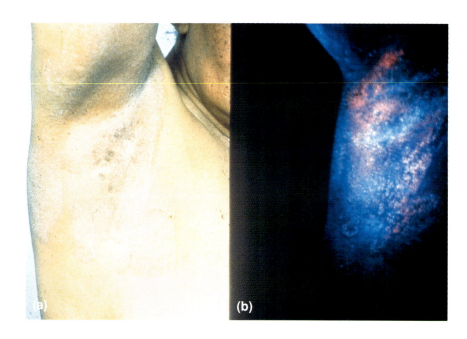

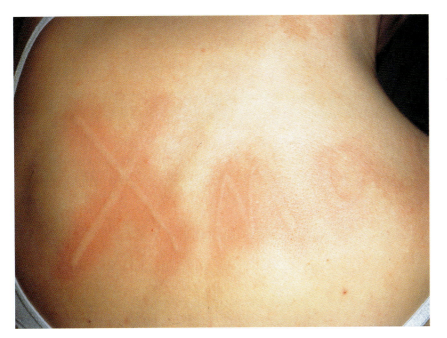

Fig. 1.25 Dermographism, showing prominent wheal-and-flare responses after stroking the skin on the upper back (the patient presented a few days before Christmas).

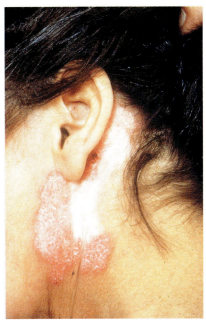

Fig. 1.26 Lupus vulgaris, a form of tuberculosis of the skin, showing a granulomatous, reddish plaque, with scarring and post-inflammatory hypopigmentation.

Prenatal diagnosis of inheritable skin diseases is a rapidly developing field and molecular biology techniques, presently used in research, will become the routine laboratory tests of the future.

There are a number of simple bedside investigations which may confirm the clinical diagnosis. These include the use of a Wood's light, collection of skin scrapings and nail clippings for mycology (Chapter 5), dermographic testing, diascopy, the extraction of the *Acarus* mite in scabies, and urine testing.

Wood's light

A Wood's light emits long-wave ultraviolet light in the 320–365nm range of the spectrum. The light should be switched on a few minutes before use and the patient should be examined in a darkened room to allow any fluorescence to be seen.

In tinea capitis (Fig. 1.23), lesions due to *Microsporum canis* and *M. audouini* show a brilliant green fluorescence, while those due to *Trichophyton schoenleinii* fluoresce with a dull green colour. Erythrasma (Fig. 1.24), caused by *Corynebacterium minitissimus*, produces a characteristic coral-pink colour, usually in the axillae or groin region. Pityriasis versicolor may be detected by the observation of pale-yellow fluorescence and the Wood's light may allow one to see lesions on the trunk which are not clinically apparent.

Wood's light can also be used to determine the depth of melanin in the skin. Variations in epidermal pigmentation are easier to see under Wood's light than in visible light (as in vitiligo or the ash-leaf macules of tuberous sclerosis). However, dermal pigmentation changes are less obvious under Wood's light (as in a blue naevus).

Testing for dermographism

Symptomatic dermographism is the most common form of physical urticaria, the physical urticarias representing around 10% of all cases of urticaria. In such patients and sometimes in patients with other forms of urticaria, brisk stroking of the skin produces a wheal-and-flare response (Fig. 1.25). The most reliable site for testing is the upper back and an itchy, palpable response usually develops after 5–10 min, although it can take longer.

Most doctors use the blunt end of a pen to stroke the skin but one may use a dermographometer which can be adjusted to apply graded pressures to the skin. The term dermographism should not be confused with white dermographism, which is the line of pallor achieved by stroking the skin in patients with atopic dermatitis and other disorders in which the skin may be erythrodermic.

Diascopy

Diascopy is a simple procedure which is used less by younger dermatologists than in the past, when cutaneous tuberculosis was more prevalent. By placing a glass slide firmly on the skin, the exclusion of blood can reveal the nature of dermal changes. Diascopy is of especial use in detecting granulomatous nodules, as in lupus vulgaris (Fig. 1.26).

The 'Acarus hunt'

Early on in my dermatology training, this endearing term conjured up images of the doctor searching for the scabies mite, armed with a monocle, shield and spear! I have since discovered that a number of implements may be used to seek out the Acarus, *Sarcoptes scabiei*. Careful exploration with a sterile needle of a scabies burrow, often in a finger web (Fig. 1.27), may reveal the female mite clinging to the needle near the tip.

Even when a diagnosis of scabies is strongly suspected from the history, morphology and distribution of the lesions, it is often difficult to find a linear burrow. The medial aspects of the feet may have been spared from excoriation. If no burrow is found one may use a fine blade (a Gillette or scalpel blade) to perform a shave

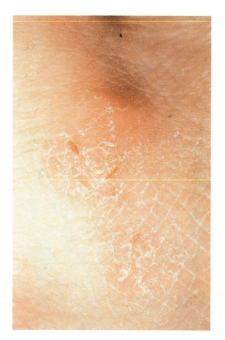

Fig. 1.27 Scabies, showing a linear burrow adjacent to a finger web.

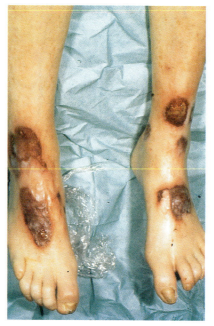

Fig. 1.28 Diabetic ulcers, occurring on the feet and ankles in an elderly woman, a localizing factor being trauma from her shoes.

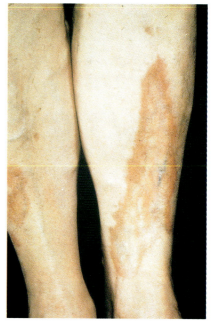

Fig. 1.29 Necrobiosis lipoidica, showing reddish-yellow atrophic plaques on the shins.

biopsy of a papule, ideally one which is not exco-riated. A local anaesthetic is usually not required and the occurrence of pinpoint bleeding demon-strates the correct depth of the procedure. Several shave samples may be placed on a microscope slide, covered with immersion oil and examined under low power. In this way, one may see a scabies mite, eggs and faeces. Immersion oil is preferred to potassium hydroxide since the latter dissolves the faeces.

Alternatively, application of immersion oil or potassium hydroxide to an affected interdigital space, followed by light scraping with a scalpel blade, may reveal the beast and its eggs.

Urine testing

Routine urine testing in dermatology patients is worth doing only if positive findings are acted upon, for instance by alerting the family practi-tioner. The finding of glycosuria and sometimes the subsequent diagnosis of diabetes mellitus is relatively common. Proteinuria or the detection of blood in the urine is less frequent. The decision to test the urine will often be directed by the clin-ical assessment of the patient.

It is wise to consider the possibility of diabetes mellitus in all patients with leg ulcers, particularly those in whom the ulceration occurs on sites subjected to pressure, such as the heels and dorsa of the feet (Fig. 1.28). Granuloma annulare is associated with diabetes in only around 5% of cases, whereas diabetes mellitus occurs in over 50% of patients with necrobiosis lipoidica, which may precede the development of diabetes (Fig. 1.29). One usually checks for glycosuria in patients with recurrent boils (furuncles) but the finding of diabetes is much less common than in patients who present with a carbuncle (a large pus-filled cavity with multiple heads). A number of the more serious skin disorders may be treated with systemic corticosteroids and regular testing of the urine for glycosuria is standard practice.

In patients with cutaneous vasculitis (often presenting with palpable purpuric lesions on the legs; Fig. 1.30), a fresh urine sample should be examined for protein, red cells and casts. A posi-

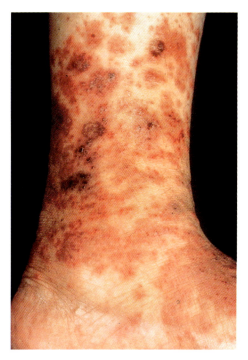

Fig. 1.30 Vasculitis, showing reddish palpable purpuric lesions and ulceration on the lower leg.

tive finding would suggest that the skin pathology is part of a systemic disease. Wood's light may be used to detect urinary (or faecal) porphyrins in patients with porphyria cutanea tarda.

In conclusion, the sound clinical assessment of the dermatology patient is an important prerequi-site to good patient care. A careful history and examination of the patient will allow a diagnosis to be made in most cases. With less common skin disorders, an appropriate differential diagnosis based on the clinical assessment will help the doctor to decide which clinical investigations should be performed.

FURTHER READING

Archer CB and Robertson SJ. *Black and White Skin Diseases: An Atlas and Text*. Blackwell Science, Oxford, 1995.

Arndt KA, Leboit PE, Robinson KJ and Wintroub BU (eds). *Cutaneous Medicine and Surgery*. WB Saunders, Philadelphia, 1995.

Champion RH, Burton JL and Ebling FJG. In: Rook A, Wilkinson DS and Ebling FJG (eds) *Textbook of Dermatology*, 5th edn. Blackwell Science, Oxford, 1992.

Fitzpatrick TB, Eisen AZ, Wolff K, Freedberg IM and Austen FK. (eds) *Dermatology in General Medicine*. Blackwell Science, Cambridge, USA, 1993.

Mitchell Sams W Jr and Lynch PJ. (eds) *Principles and Practice of Dermatology*. Churchill Livingstone, New York, 1990.

Chapter 2

Dermatopathology

Rino Cerio

Because the skin is easily accessible to biopsy, microscopic examination has always been especially important to the dermatologist and is often needed to make a definite diagnosis. Dermatopathology is continuing to evolve as a medical specialty. This chapter will explore what can be learnt by examining skin samples, prepared in a variety of ways, with the microscope. Investigation of hair and nails is covered in Chapters 7 and 8.

For the most effective results, when examining skin biopsy sections, it is essential that clinicians provide detailed information, including age, sex, skin type, exact site, clinical history and description of the skin disorder including, where possible, a differential diagnosis. Clinicians should know of the practical importance of proper selection of skin lesions for pathological examination, the required depth and the preparation necessary for optimum processing of the specimen. They should also have some knowledge of potential artefacts, the scope and value of special stains, both tinctorial and immunohistochemical, and how electron microscopy can help. These areas, in addition to discussion of how to interpret a histopathology report, will be covered in this chapter.

SELECTION OF SKIN BIOPSY SITE

The selection of the skin biopsy site obviously depends on the type of lesion. There are five main reasons why a skin biopsy may be required:

- Excision of epidermal or dermal neoplasm, whether benign or malignant. Excision margins are required.
- An incision biopsy for confirmation of a similar lesion which is too big for removal and will be treated by alternative methods, for example, more complex surgery, radiotherapy or cryotherapy. This is most useful for basal cell carcinoma or *in situ* squamous cell carcinoma (Bowen's disease) but should be avoided in melanocytic lesions, particularly if malignant melanoma is suspected, where the overall morphology is desirable for diagnosis.

- An incision biopsy of a skin eruption which is difficult to categorize. Most will be inflammatory but sometimes cutaneous T-cell lymphoma is suspected. In these instances two or three biopsies may be submitted for examination.
- Fresh tissue incision skin biopsies can be taken for immunopathological study, especially immunofluorescence when investigating suspected autoimmune dermatoses, for example, bullous pemphigoid, vasculitis or lupus erythematosus (LE). Perilesional samples will yield positive results in blistering dermatoses whereas in discoid LE lesional skin is required. A lupus band test may help to confirm a diagnosis of systemic LE; the biopsy is usually taken from non-sun-exposed skin. Dividing the biopsy longitudinally by half – parallel biopsy – will provide material for routine histology and fresh frozen tissue (Fig. 2.1).
- Parallel or adjacent incision biopsies may be required and fresh tissue sent to the microbiologist when infection is suspected. The tissue can be cultured for various organisms, including atypical mycobacteria and deep fungi, or examined for protozoa or filarial worms.

SKIN BIOPSY TECHNIQUES

Six biopsy techniques are currently employed under local anaesthetic (Table 2.1). The specimens are placed in formalin for routine paraffin processing, Michel's medium or liquid nitrogen for immunofluorescence studies or a sterile pot for microbiological tests. Laboratory personnel who perform electron micropsy and cell culture usually participate in the handling of a freshly obtained specimen.

WHEN SHOULD SKIN BIOPSY BE AVOIDED?

For the most part, the aim of skin biopsy is to obtain diagnostic information. However, the question of when or where biopsy samples are

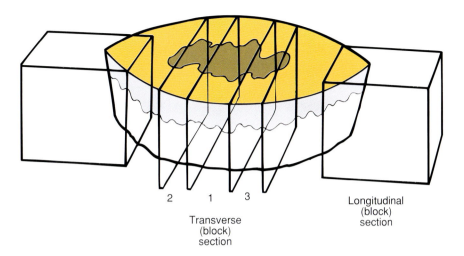

Fig. 2.1a Excision of tumour: transverse and longitudinal tissue blocks are removed at macroscopic examination to provide appropriate sections.

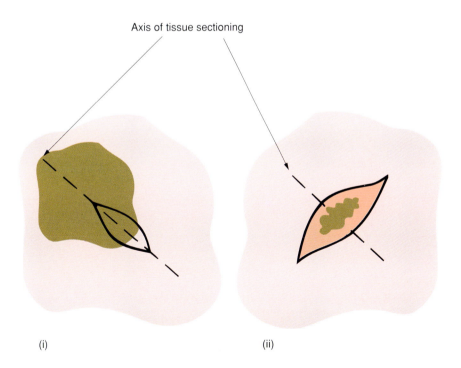

Fig. 2.1b Tissue sectioning for routine haematoxylin and eosin staining, showing (i) longitudinal sectioning of an elliptical incision biopsy of a rash and (ii) transverse sectioning of an excised skin tumour.

21

carried out is vital to achieving a successful outcome. Some clinical circumstances can hinder diagnostic dermatopathology. For example, when the clinical distinction between psoriasis is difficult, the histopathological features may be reported as those of eczematous psoriasis or psoriasiform dermatitis, and a biopsy of florid granuloma annulare from the lower leg may be impossible to distinguish from necrobiosis lipoidica. There are circumstances when skin biopsy is best avoided, unless absolutely essential (Table 2.2).

PREPARATION OF HISTOPATHOLOGICAL SECTIONS

Fixation

Most laboratories use some variant of formaldehyde (4%), often with saline, to fix skin biopsies for at least 2 h. The specimen is described macroscopically and given an accession number after checking the specimen, pot and request form for errors. Only larger specimens require trimming. It is important to realize that the macroscopic description is an important part of the overall

Table 2.1 Skin biopsy techniques	
Excision	For removal of a single lesion. An elliptical or fusiform-shaped area of skin is removed
Incision biopsy (wedge)	Similar to excision but narrower; to include fat in suspected panniculitis. Some normal perilesional skin is included for comparison
Punch biopsy	(3–4 mm) Useful if tissue available is limited but accurate sample is essential. A rapid procedure, sometimes useful in children
Curettage	For hyperkeratotic lesions, e.g. seborrhoeic keratoses, viral warts, basal cell carcinomas. Usually accompanied by cautery
Shave biopsy	For protuberant facial lesions, e.g. benign intradermal naevi
Snip	For skin tags; also for onchocerciasis

Table 2.2 Skin biopsy is best avoided in these circumstances unless essential	
Infants	Although local anaesthetic creams or gels make this easier
Upper trunk	In order to avoid keloid formation
Lower legs in elderly patients	Poor healing may occur
Cardiac patients	Valvular disease means there is a potential risk of subacute bacterial endocarditis (debatable) Aspirin/anticoagulants can produce extensive bleeding
Patients with HIV or hepatitis B	In order to minimize cross-infection
Melanoma incision	Primary excision is preferable as it has been argued that incision, particularly punch biopsy, may disseminate tumour cells

histopathology report, not only in order to identify details of material received and what was processed, but also for medico-legal reasons. Excision specimens can be marked with Indian ink and divided into one or more 4-mm blocks transversely. If necessary, two lateral blocks can also be examined (Fig. 2.1). Fixatives which are commonly used include:

- *10% Formal saline*
  Formalin = (40% formaldehyde) 100 ml
  Sodium chloride 8–5 g
  Tap water 900 ml
- *Buffered 10% formalin (pH 7.0)*
  Formalin = (40% formaldehyde) 100 ml
  Sodium dihydrogen orthophosphate
  ($NaH_2PO_4H_2O$) 4 g
  Disodium hydrogen orthophosphate
  anhydrous Na_2HPO_4) 6.5 g
  Tap water 900 ml
- *FMA*
  Formalin (40% formaldehyde) 100 ml
  Mercuric chloride 20 g
  Glacial acetic acid 30 ml
  Distilled water 900 ml
- *Michel's medium*
  1. Ammonium sulphate 55 g in 100 ml buffer
  2. Buffer – 2.5 ml 1 mol/L potassium citrate (pH 7)
  5 ml 0.1 mol/L magnesium sulphate
  5 ml 0.1 N ethyl maleimide
  87.5 ml distilled water
  (1 and 2) mixed with 1 mol/L potassium hydroxide to pH 7.0

Specimens for immunofluorescence studies can be snap-frozen in liquid nitrogen and transported to the cryostat for sectioning, or transported in Michel's medium, which preserves immunoreactants for several weeks. Specimens for microbiology have to be placed in a sterile container and delivered to the laboratory immediately.

Routine paraffin processing

Formaldehyde-fixed material is passed through graded (50–100%) alcohol to become dehydrated, then two to three changes of xylene or chloroform to become defatted (cleared) and finally, through two or three changes of paraffin at 60 °C. The entire process, which is fully automated, requires 24 h. Shorter cycles are also possible for small biopsies. Embedding the material is the most important stage and, if the epidermis is not recognized, orientation will be far from ideal, making interpretation difficult.

Tissue sectioning

The surface of the skin must end up at a 90° angle to the knife when the tissue block is mounted on a microtome and sections cut are usually 5 µm thick. Often several step sections or levels are made available for examination. If necessary, deeper cuts are performed into or throughout the block.

For routine haematoxylin and eosin staining, an elliptical incision biopsy of a rash is usually sectioned longitudinally. This allows comparison between lesional and adjacent normal-appearing skin. The histological appearance of the skin varies at different body sites, particularly with regard to epidermal thickness. Hence, it is only by comparing lesional epidermis with non-lesional epidermis that a pathologist can confidently refer to acanthosis (thickening of the epidermis), as seen, for example, in eczema, psoriasis and lichen planus.

Following excision of a skin tumour, the specimen is usually cut transversely. This enables the pathologist to comment on the lateral margins of excision, and further sections may be taken if deemed necessary. The general principles of tissue sectioning are illustrated in Figure 2.1b.

Special stains

Most histopathological diagnoses can be made by routine haematoxylin and eosin staining. A number of special stains are also valuable when used appropriately (Table 2.3).

Artefacts

The dermatologist may be misled by a number of

Table 2.3 Some tinctorial stains used in dermatology

Special stains	Tissue constituent	Appearance
Periodic acid–Schiff (PAS)	Glycogen	Magenta red (diastase-sensitive)
	Mucopolysaccharides	Red (fungal wall red)
van Gieson	Collagen	Red
	Muscle	Yellow
	Nerve	
Congo red	Amyloid	Red with green birefringence
Acid Orcein–Giemsa	Elastic fibre	Dark brown
	Collagen	Pink
	Melanin	Black
	Haemosiderin	Green/yellow
	Amyloid	Light blue
	Mast cell granules	Purple
Masson's trichrome	Collagen	Green
	Muscle + fibrin	Red
Aldehyde fuchsin	Elastic fibre	Purple
Gomori's	Reticulin	Black
Alcian blue (pH 4.5/0.5)	Acid mucopolysaccharides	Blue
Toluidine blue	(AMPS)	Metachromatic purple, including mast cells
Perls' Prussian blue	Iron (haemosiderin)	Blue
Masson's Fontana	Melanin	Black
Von Kossa	Calcium salts	Brown/black
Grocott's methenamine silver	Fungal wall	Black
Gram	Bacteria	Gram + ve blue/violet
		Gram – ve red/pink
Fite-Frac	Acid-fast bacilli	Red

pitfalls (see Table 2.4). Apart from those resulting from the biopsy procedure or tissue processing, artefacts can arise *in vivo*, unrelated to skin disease *per se*. These include artefacts arising from medicaments and physical influences such as excoriation, friction, injections, electric current and sunburn. The dermatopathologist's ability to identify specific changes will be of value for the clinician in obscure cases.

Tzanck smear

Tzanck smears are still useful to confirm herpes skin infection (Fig 2.2) or suspected pemphigus vulgaris. Bullae should be new and not infected with bacteria. The roof is removed and the floor scraped with a scalpel. The sample is then spread on to a glass slide, air-dried or fixed by immersion 4–5 times in 95% ethyl alcohol. The best stain is Giemsa, which requires only 2–3 min.

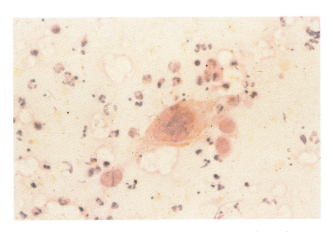

Fig. 2.2 Tzanck smear showing herpes-infected keratinocytes.

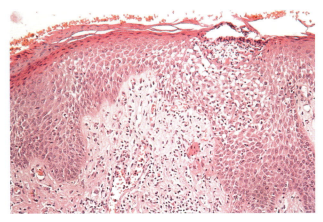

Fig. 2.3 Eczematous tissue reaction (spongiotic dermatitis). There is spongiosis in the epidermis, accompanied by a superficial perivascular infiltrate.

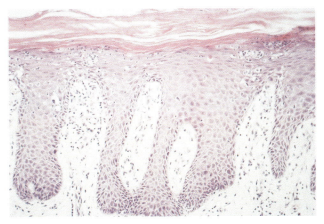

Fig. 2.4 Psoriasiform tissue reaction, as seen in psoriasis, showing psoriasiform hyperplasia of the epidermis, absence of the granular layer and para-keratosis.

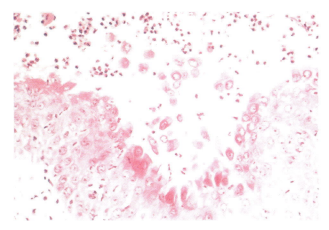

Fig. 2.5 Pemphigus vulgaris, showing suprabasal clefting and separation, with clumps of acantholytic epidermal cells.

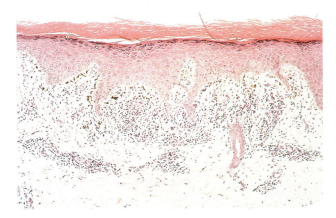

Fig. 2.6 Lichen planus, showing a band-like infiltrate, hyper-keratosis and hypergranulosis.

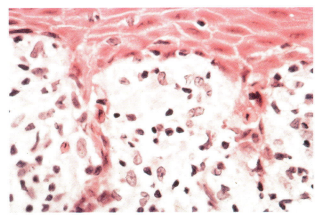

Fig. 2.7 Lichen planus, a lichenoid interface dermatitis, obscuring the dermal–epidermal interface with acanthosis and colloid body formation.

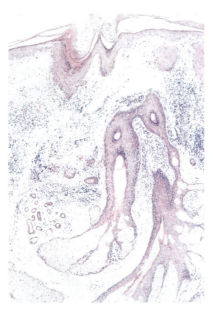

Fig. 2.8 Discoid lupus erythematosus, a quiet interface dermatitis with superficial and deep perivascular and periappendageal lymphohistiocytic infiltration, epidermal atrophy, follicular plugging and focal liquefaction degeneration of the basal layer.

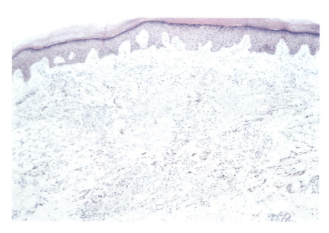

Fig. 2.9 Granuloma annulare, showing a well-demarcated focus of collagen degeneration in the dermis, surrounded by a predominantly histiocytic infiltrate.

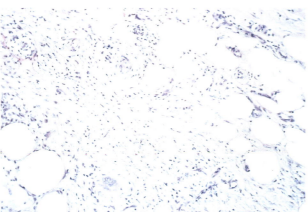

Fig. 2.10 Erythema nodosum, showing a chronic inflammatory infiltrate extending from an interlobular septum into a subcutaneous fat lobule.

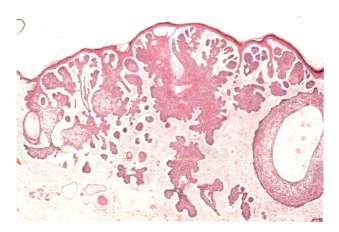

Fig. 2.11 Basal cell carcinoma, showing dermal basophilic tumour islands with appendageal differentiation.

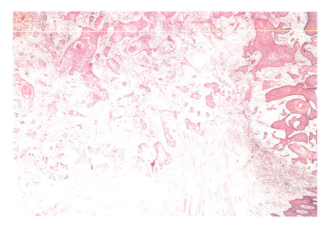

Fig. 2.12 Squamous cell carcinoma, arising in the epidermis and invading deeply into the dermis.

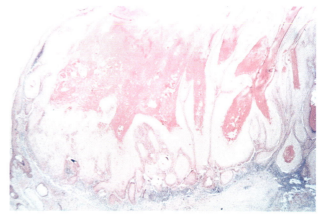

Fig. 2.13 Keratoacanthoma with central keratin plug and 'ground glass' cytoplasm.

Table 2.4 Potential dermatopathological artefacts

Poor orientation confusing true epidermal and papillary dermis appearance

Formaldehyde fixation vacuolation of epidermis

Scratch marks across tissue due to nick in microtome knife

Tissue carried over from microtome knife

Foreign bodies, e.g. formaldehyde pigments, suture, alternaria, spores, starch

Polarization of cell nuclear material by electric current in curetted specimens

Clumped mitoses in podophyllin-treated warts

Pyknotic prickle cells from methotrexate or hydroxy-urea-treated patients

Microscopic examination can be immediate. In herpes, multinucleate giant cells and inclusion bodies are seen. In pemphigus, acantholytic cells can be observed. Further subclassification is not possible.

COMMON HISTOPATHOLOGICAL PATTERNS

A knowledge of some of the common histopathological patterns of skin disorders may improve the clinician's diagnostic ability.

Rashes

As discussed in Chapter 1, if the diagnosis is not obvious from the morphology and distribution of an eruption, one should consider which level of the skin is predominantly involved by the pathological process.

Disorders with epidermal change include the various types of eczema (dermatitis/eczematous dermatitis), psoriasis and the immunobullous disorders, in which there is abnormal cellular cohesion either within the epidermis (as in pemphigus vulgaris) or between the epidermis and the dermis (as in bullous pemphigoid). An

eczematous tissue reaction (Fig. 2.3), with superficial perivascular infiltration and spongiosis of the epidermis (the histopathological precursor of vesiculation) is seen, for example, in allergic contact dermatitis, in which a biopsy is not usually necessary. In a **psoriasiform tissue reaction** (Fig 2.4), the main features are supra-papillary exudate (containing oedema and often neutrophils), with focal parakeratosis and psoriasiform hyperplasia of the epidermis. In pemphigus vulgaris, there is suprabasal clefting and separation, with clumps of acantholytic cells (Fig. 2.5).

An **interface dermatitis** can be considered an example of a superficial perivascular dermatitis (as in lichen planus (Fig. 2.6) or erythema multiforme) or superficial and deep perivascular dermatitis (as in discoid LE). In lichen planus, there is a dense band-like, **lichenoid** infiltrate in the papillary dermis, which can obscure the dermal–epidermal interface (Fig. 2.7). In discoid LE (Fig. 2.8), there is superficial and deep lymphohistiocytic infiltration, with atrophy of the epidermis, follicular plugging and focal liquefaction degeneration of the basal layer. In erythema multiforme, there is relatively little inflammatory cell infiltration, the predominant feature being **vacuolar** alteration of the basal layer of the epidermis.

Dermal changes are seen in a number of skin diseases, including granuloma annulare (Fig. 2.9) and lymphomas. Inflammatory disorders of the subcutaneous fat tend to be persistent. There are various forms of panniculitis, erythema nodosum (Fig. 2.10) being an example of a septal (rather than lobular) panniculitis.

Skin tumours

Common skin tumours include basal cell epithelioma (basal cell carcinoma), squamous cell carcinoma and keratoacanthoma. A basal cell carcinoma (Fig. 2.11) is composed of islands of uniform basophilic cells, arising from basal keratinocytes, which form epidermal buds with eventual dermal invasion. Squamous cell carcinoma (Fig. 2.12), derived from moderately well-

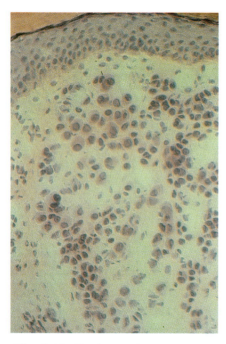

Fig. 2.14 Benign melanocytic naevus, with mono-morphic dermal nests.

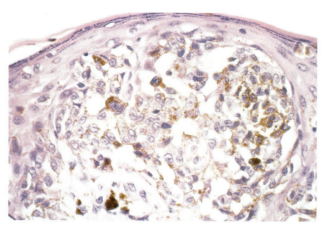

Fig. 2.15 Malignant melanoma destroying the epidermis.

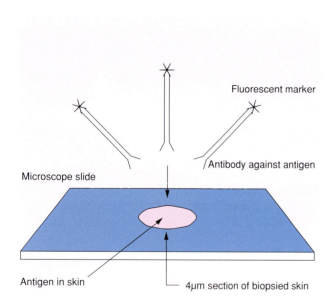

Fig. 2.16 Direct immunofluorescence. Fluorescein-labelled antihuman immunoglobulin G will bind to immunoglobulin G deposits along the basement membrane zone in bullous pemphigoid.

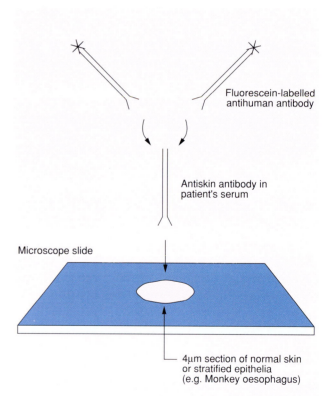

Fig. 2.17 Indirect immunofluorescence: fluorescing antibodies are used to label where antibodies in a patient's serum are bound to normal skin *in vitro*.

differentiated keratinocytes, destroys the dermal–epidermal junction and invades the dermis in an irregular way. Histologically, a keratoacanthoma (Fig. 2.13), may resemble a squamous cell carcinoma, but the overall architecture is more symmetrical, as there is a regular rim or shoulder.

The histopathological diagnosis of malignant melanoma is not always obvious. Characteristic examples of a benign melanocytic naevus (Fig. 2.14), is a superficial spreading malignant melanoma and a nodular malignant melanoma (Fig. 2.15) are shown here to complement the clinical descriptions given in Chapter 1.

IMMUNOPATHOLOGICAL TECHNIQUES

Cutaneous immunopathology has added exciting new dimensions to diagnostic dermatopathology. Special stains can differentiate certain subcomponents of the skin but it is the routine use of antibodies and immunocytochemistry in identifying specific antigens that has been a real advance. The application of such techniques is most valuable in the diagnosis of autoimmune bullous disorders, vasculitis, LE and subcutaneous neoplasms. However, few, if any, immunological patterns are disease-specific. The extent to which cutaneous immunopathology aids diagnosis depends upon the problems posed by an individual specimen. Immunopathological techniques are only useful when combined with routine light microscopy and clinical information.

Immunofluorescence

DIRECT AND INDIRECT IMMUNOFLUORESCENCE

Most histopathologists tend to use direct (Fig. 2.16) and indirect immunofluorescence (Fig. 2.17) and immunocytochemical techniques. **Direct immunofluorescence** is a method for *in situ* demonstration of antibody in tissue, whereas **indirect immunofluorescence** is a serological technique employed to demonstrate and quantify the amount of circulating antibody.

Table 2.5 Direct immunofluorescence in autoimmune blistering diseases

Disease	Pattern and nature of immunoreactants
Pemphigus	Epidermal cell surface deposits of IgG and C3
Bullous pemphigoid	Linear, homogeneous deposits of IgG (epidermal side on salt split skin) and C3 at the dermal–epidermal junction
Linear IgA dermatosis	Linear homogeneous deposits of IgA at the dermal–epidermal junction
Herpes (pemphigoid) gestationis	Linear homogeneous deposits of C3 at the dermal–epidermal junction
Epidermolysis bullosa acquisita	Linear homogeneous deposits of IgG (dermal side on salt split skin) and C3 at the dermal–epidermal junction
Cicatricial pemphigoid	Linear homogeneous deposits of IgG and C3 at the dermal–epidermal junction
Dermatitis herpetiformis	Focal granular deposits of IgA at the papillary tips
Intradermal neutrophilic IgA	Epidermal cell-surface deposits of IgA
Bullous eruption of lupus erythematosus	Linear homogeneous, or linear systemic non-homogeneous deposits of multiple immunoglobulins, C3 and fibrin at the dermal–epidermal junction

IgA = Immunoglobulin A.

Any disease in which there is a deposition of immunoglobulins or other substances in specific sites or patterns can be diagnosed by immunofluorescence. However, over the years, due to better positive yields immunofluorescence has been employed on cryostat sections (with and without incubation in Michel's transport medium) to identify tissue-bound autoantibodies, C3 and fibrin by direct method (Table 2.5). In addition, by using normal skin as a substrate, autoantibody directed against cutaneous components can be detected by testing the patient's serum by indirect immunofluorescence.

Titres are of practical value in assessing disease activity in patients with pemphigus vulgaris and, arguably, bullous pemphigoid (Fig. 2.18). The technique is easy to perform but requires the expense of a fluorescence microscope.

SALT SPLIT IMMUNOFLUORESCENCE

As several subepidermal blistering conditions have similar light and immunofluorescence findings, it may be necessary to develop more sophisticated methods to distinguish them. Normal human skin incubated in 1 mol/L sodium chloride for 48–72 h results in a split at the level of the lamina lucida. Bullous pemphigoid antibodies bind to the epidermal side (roof) and the floor of the blister in bullous pemphigoid, whereas epidermolysis bullosa acquisita antibodies bind solely to the dermal side (floor) of the split skin. This technique is more sensitive and can also be used to identify low titres of circulating immunoglobulin A and G antibodies in cicatricial pemphigoid. Even if circulating antibodies are not present, utilization of direct immunofluorescence evaluation of perilesional skin exposure to salt-splitting in the same way can demonstrate *in situ* bound immunoreactants.

ANTIGENIC MAPPING

Light microscopy cannot distinguish between junctional and dermolytic forms of epidermolysis. Both appear as non-inflammatory subepidermal blisters. Electron microscopy will show the exact plane of blistering. Alternatively, immunofluorescence labelling with type IV collagen, laminin and bullous pemphigoid antisera can be used to locate cleavage on fresh frozen tissue (Fig. 2.19). This method can also be used to show altered antigenicity of the basement membrane zone, for example, type VII collagen, kalinin and uncein in several subsets of junctional dystrophic epidermolysis bullosa (Chapter 3; Table 2.5).

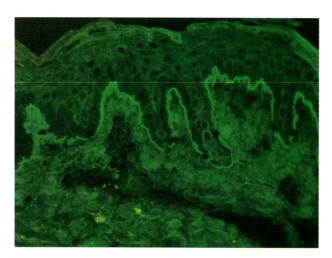

Fig. 2.18a Indirect immunofluorescence demonstrating positive circulating autoantibody in bullous pemphigoid at a titre of 1:80.

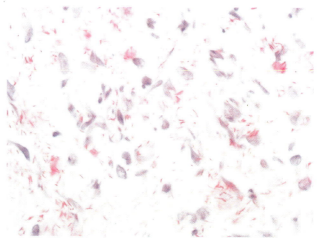

Fig. 2.18b Numerous acid-fast bacillus-positive *Mycobacterium leprae* in histiocytoid lepromatous leprosy.

Immunocytochemistry

In immunocytochemistry, antibodies are used to identify antigens and tissue structures. These cell markers are visualized by attaching peroxidase or avidin–biotin complex to the antibody, which may be mono- or polyclonal.

Immunocytochemical methods using peroxidase or avidin–biotin conjugated monoclonal or polyclonal antibodies tend to be employed for routine paraffin sections. In this way a permanent labelled section is produced with superior morphology to that seen in cryostat sections. Depending on the individual case, an altered panel of cell markers, both monoclonal and polyclonal, is now commercially available (Fig. 2.20). The applications of immunocytochemistry in

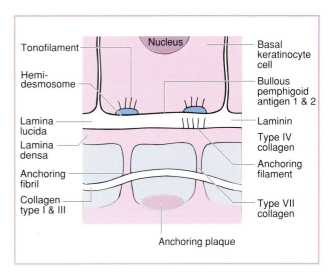

Fig. 2.19 Diagrammatic representation of basement membrane zone.

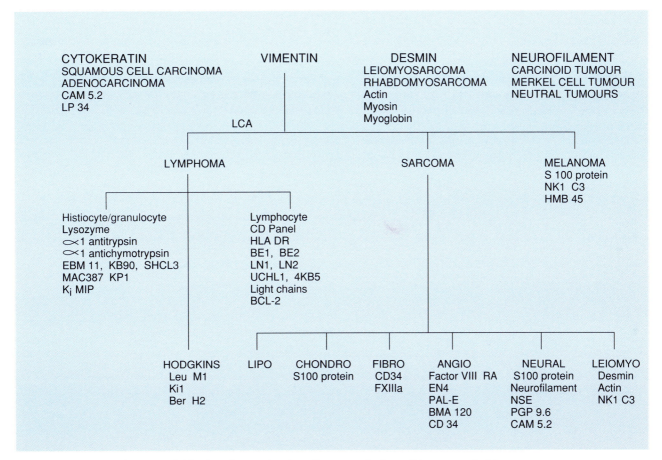

Fig. 2.20 Cell markers useful in the diagnosis of malignant spindle-cell tumours of skin.

Table 2.6 Skin infections diagnosed by histology

BACTERIAL SKIN INFECTIONS

Gram-positive

Cocci	Impetigo	*Streptococcus pyogenes* group A (rarely B, C, or G) *Staphylococcus aureus*
Bacilli (AFB+)	Granuloma Millary tuberculosis Lepromatous leprosy Atypical	*Mycobacterium tuberculosis* *M. leprae* (Fig. 2.18b) *M. marinum* (Fig. 2.19), *ulcerans, kansasii, fortuitum, chelonei* and *avium intracellulare*
(AFB+/-)	Madura foot	*Nocardia madurae*
(AFB-)	Anthrax Erythrasma Acne	*Bacillus anthracis* *Corynebacterium minutissimum* (coral-red fluorescence) *Propionibacterium acnes*

Gram-negative

Cocci	Ulcer	*Neisseria gonorrhoeae*
Bacilli	Chancroid Granuloma inguinale Green ulcer Bacillary angiomatosis	*Haemophilus ducreyi* *Calymmatobacterium granulomatis* *Pseudomonas aeruginosa* *Bartonella henselae, B. quintana*
Spirochaetes	Erythema chronicum migrans Yaws Syphilis	*Borrelia burgdorferi* *Treponema pertenue* *Treponema pallidum* } dark-ground illumination

FUNGAL SKIN INFECTIONS

Yeast-like	*Candida albicans* (Fig. 2.20), *Pityrosporum orbiculare*
Yeasts	*Actinomyces israelii* (Gram + ive; Fig. 2.21) *Cryptococcus neoformans*
Dermatophytes	*Trichophyton rubrum* (Fig. 2.22), *mentagrophytes, interdigitale, schoenleinii, verrucosum* *Microsporum canis* *Epidermophyton floccosum*
Dimorphic fungi	*Histoplasma capsulatum* (within macrophages) *Blastomyces dermatitidis* *Coccidioides immitis* *Sporothrix schenkii* Chromomycosis (Fig. 2..23)

Table 2.6 continues

VIRAL SKIN INFECTIONS

Viral subtype	Group	Skin diseases
DNA	Pox	Molluscum contagiosum
		Orf
	Herpes	Simplex types I and II
		Zoster
		Cytomegalovirus
		Human B-cell lymphotrophic virus
	Papova	Human papillomavirus
RNA	Picorna	Coxsackie virus groups A + B
	Paramyxo	Measles
	Toga	Rubella (German measles)
	Retro	Human immunodeficiency virus (HTLV 3) HTLV I

SKIN INFESTATIONS

Scabies		*Sarcoptes scabiei*
Demodex		*Demodex folliculorum*
Threadworms		*Enterobius vermicularis*
Larva migrans		*Strongyloides stercoralis*
Onchocerciasis		*Onchocerca volvulus* (Fig. 2.24)
Leishmaniasis (via sandfly)		*Leishmania tropica* (protozoa-filled macrophages

AFB = Acid-fast bacillus; HTLV = human T-cell lymphotrophic virus.

dermatology are summarized in Tables 2.5 and 2.6.

HISTOPATHOLOGY AND SKIN INFECTIONS

Skin infections remain common in clinical practice, especially in susceptible individuals, and may present to any practitioner in all fields of medicine. There is a broad spectrum of infective skin disorders which can be diagnosed by histology, although histopathological examination may not be essential for the diagnosis to be made. Susceptible patients include paediatric, geriatric, diabetic, immunosuppressed individuals and immigrants. Bacterial and fungal infections are also discussed in Chapter 5 and the Tzanck smear for the confirmation of herpes infection has been described above. Table 2.6 and Figs 2.18b, 2.21-7 shows some of the more easily demonstrated infections.

ELECTRON MICROSCOPY

In recent years the electron microscope has become less practical as a dermatological diagnostic tool and has been superseded by newer pathology techniques, such as immunocytochemistry, especially immunomapping of the basement membrane zone. However, it is often readily available and can be useful to both the dermatopathologists and dermatologists. Some situations are outlined in Table 2.7.

THE HISTOPATHOLOGY REPORT

Dermatology is riddled with synonyms and curious names describing disease processes. Similarly, dermatopathology adds a further confusing established nomenclature to an already complicated subject. Consequently, there is much to be said for providing clinicians with a descriptive report that is understood by both the pathologist and the clinician. When possible, the pathologist should offer a differential diagnosis rather than the commonly used term: 'non-specific pathological features seen'. This is especially true for inflammatory dermatoses.

Continuing communication between physician and pathologist is often essential. This can best be achieved by regular review meetings to discuss difficult cases.

Table 2.7 Electron microscopic applications in dermatology

Infection – herpesvirus, orf, human papillomavirus

Disturbed keratinization, e.g. epidermolytic hyperkeratosis

Disturbed pigmentation, e.g. amelanotic melanoma

Blister formation – prenatal diagnosis of epidermolysis bullosa

Undifferentiated tumours – metastasis, Merkel cell tumours, carcinoid tumour (Fig. 2.28) histiocytoses

Storage diseases – mucopolysaccharidoses

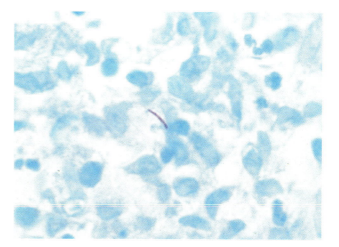

Fig. 2.21 Atypical *Mycobacterium marinum* from fish tank granuloma.

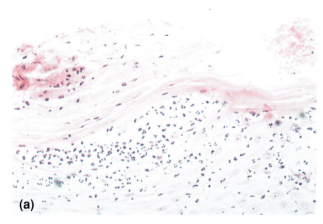

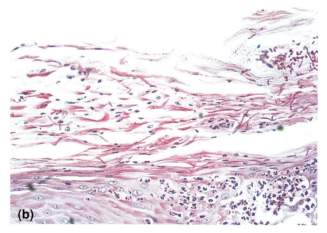

Fig. 2.22a,b Positive periodic acid–Schiff *Candida albicans* invisible on haematoxylin and eosin staining.

Courtesy of N. Ramnarain and G. Orchard, St John's Institute of Dermatology, London.

Skin sampling in certain cases can be far from ideal, because of the nature of the biopsy, the biopsy site, modification by therapy, modification of external complicating factors, such as excoriation and infection, or the biopsy may not represent the disease process as a whole. Clearly, in these circumstances the dermatopathologist will be unable to offer a specific diagnosis. In difficult cases, the pathologist can often refute a suspected clinical diagnosis as well as support one.

Pathologists should be encouraged to offer a carefully worded view on further management of lesions, especially in dealing with the removal of difficult skin tumours, such as malignant melanoma or other borderline melanocytic lesions. However, it should be appreciated that there is continuing debate regarding desirable margins of excision in malignant melanoma (of varying Breslow thickness) and the pathologist therefore should always be cautious not to be too dogmatic. Comments on lack of excision in reports only distract the clinician if he or she has performed a curettage or superficial (e.g. shave) biopsy intentionally. In the circumstances it is better to describe the tumour as a curettage specimen or filling the dermis and reaching the deep margins. This should avoid confusion by inappropriately using the term 'incompletely excised' when this was not the intention anyway.

Further studies may be necessary using special stains or even immunohistochemistry to exclude or confirm the morphological diagnosis. Perhaps the most important option in non-diagnostic cases is to cut further levels into the block or even to re-examine further tissue not processed for clues to diagnosis. Finally, if the dermatopathologist adopts a systematic approach using terminology understood by clinical colleagues and ensures clinicopathological cooperation and coordination, the patient will be best served, and problematic medicolegal aspects of histopathological reporting avoided.

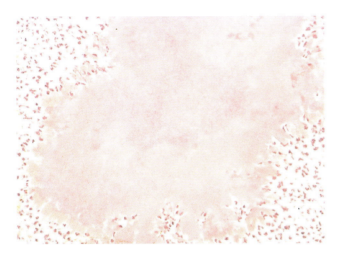

Fig. 2.23 *Actinomyces israelii* using haematoxylin and eosin staining. Courtesy of N. Ramnarain and G. Orchard, St John's Institute of Dermatology, London.

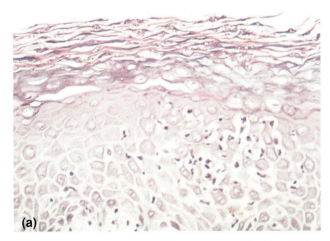

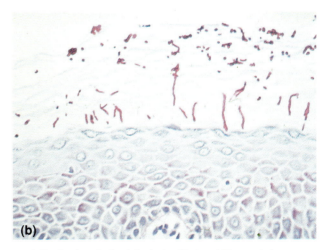

Fig. 2.24a, b *Trichophyton rubrum* identified by periodic acid-Schiff staining. Courtesy of N. Ramnarain and G. Orchard, St John's Institute of Dermatology, London.

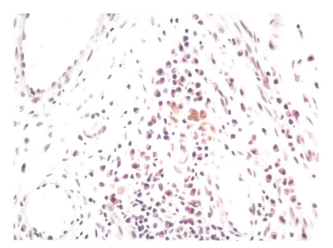

Fig. 2.25 'Copper penny' appearance in chromocycosis in superficial dermis on haematoxylin and eosin staining. Courtesy of N. Ramnarain and G. Orchard, St John's Institute of Dermatology, London.

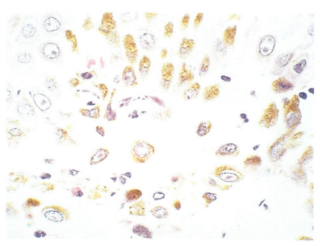

Fig. 2.26 *Onchocerca* microlarva seen in superficial dermis. Courtesy of N. Ramnarain and G. Orchard, St John's Dermatology Institute, London.

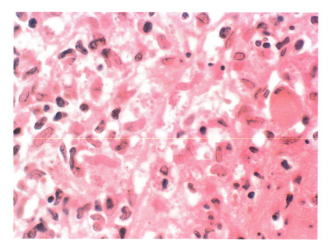

Fig. 2.27 Macrophages full of *Leishmania donovani* bodies. Courtesy of N. Ramnarain and G. Orchard, St John's Institute of Dermatology, London.

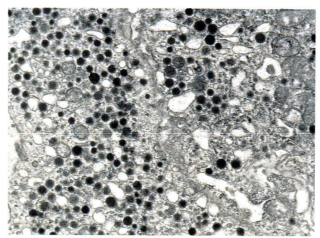

Fig. 2.28 Electron micrograph of metastatic cutaneous carcinoid tumour cell showing characteristic neurosecretory granules. Courtesy of C.B. Archer.

FURTHER READING

Arndt KA, Leboit PE, Robinson JK and Wintroub BU (eds) *Cutaneous Medicine and Surgery*, Vols 1 and 2. WB Saunders, Philadelphia, 1995.

Bancroft JD and Stevens A. *Histopathology Stains and their Diagnostic Uses*. Churchill-Livingstone, Edinburgh, 1975.

Dahl MV, Lynch PJ. *Current Opinions in Dermatology*, 2nd edn. Current Science, Philadelphia, 1995.

Drury RAB and Wallington EA. *Carlton's Histological Techniques*, 4th edn. Oxford Medical, Oxford, 1967.

Mckee PH. *Pathology of the Skin*. Gower Medical Publishing, Singapore, 1989.

Mehregan AH and Hashimoto SK. *Appleton & Lange Pinkus' Guide to Dermatopathology*, 5th edn. Prentice Hall, Connecticut, 1991.

Murphy F. *Dermatopathology*. WB Saunders, Philadelphia, 1995.

Chapter 3

General laboratory investigations

Christopher R. Lovell

■ **Specific diagnostic problems**

Pruritus
Flushing
Atopic dermatitis, urticaria and
erythroderma
  Atopic dermatitis (atopic eczema)
  Urticaria
  Erythroderma
Problems with hair and nails
  Diffuse alopecia
  Excessive hair growth
  Nail disorders
Pigmentary disorders
Blistering disorders
Photosensitivity
Purpura and vasculitis
Connective tissue diseases
  Lupus erythematosus
  Scleroderma
  Dermatomyositis
Infections
  Viral
  Bacterial
  Fungi/yeasts
  Protozoa

Metabolic disorders
  Lipid abnormalities
  Mucopolysaccharide abnormalities
  Amyloidosis
  Disorders of amino acid metabolism
  Vitamin disorders
  Ichthyoses
  Miscellaneous
Other inflammatory disorders
■ **Monitoring drugs commonly used in
dermatology**

In the typical dermatology outpatient a diagnosis is achieved by a brief, directed history, careful examination and, where appropriate, skin biopsy. A minority of patients require more detailed investigation, including blood and urine tests, which may be helpful to narrow down possible differential diagnoses, or to hint at prognosis. Even in simple clinical situations, investigation may reveal surprising results, for example, a blood count demonstrating acute leukaemia in an adult with unusually florid viral warts. In this chapter some investigations are listed which should help to elucidate common clinical problems, and perhaps unearth the odd rarity.

In practice, blood tests are more commonly performed in order to monitor therapy with potentially toxic drugs. The chapter ends with suggested protocols for commonly used agents; these are based on manufacturers' recommendations or recent reviews.

SPECIFIC DIAGNOSTIC PROBLEMS

This section examines diagnostic problems which are commonly encountered in the dermatology clinic. This is followed by suggested investigations for the patient with a connective tissue or collagen–vascular disease, suspected infection and a few rarer disorders.

Pruritus

Itching without any obvious primary dermatosis may be a presenting feature of an underlying metabolic disorder (Table 3.1). A full blood count may reveal polycythaemia, an important cause of itching after water exposure. Iron deficiency, even in the absence of anaemia, is an important cause of generalized pruritus, especially in the menstruating female. It is therefore important to check serum iron and iron-binding capacity or serum ferritin, even if the haemoglobin is normal. Liver function tests may demonstrate cholestasis, for example, due to mechanical obstruction of bile flow. Particularly in the middle-aged female, it is worth checking an autoimmune profile, consid-

ering primary biliary cirrhosis. Direct measurement of bile salts in the blood is unhelpful.

Both hyper- and hypothyroidism may underlie generalized pruritus. Diabetes is associated only with an increased incidence of genital itching. In post-menopausal pruritus, typically associated with hot flushes, plasma follicular stimulating hormone (FSH) and luteinizing hormone (LH) may be elevated. Pruritus due to uraemia is usually associated with other features of renal failure; serum urea and electrolytes and creatinine are simple screening tests. There may be secondary hyperparathyroidism. A raised caeruloplasmin may be an early sign of an underlying lymphoma.

Flushing

Flushing is due to vascular, neural or endocrine factors, or a combination of all three. Perimenopausal flushing is common; a hormonal profile should indicate perimenopausal changes.

Episodic flushing, particularly after alcohol, raises the possibility of carcinoid, justifying

Table 3.1 Investigation of unexplained pruritus	
Full blood count	?Polycythaemiavera, ?microcytosis
Serum iron/total iron-binding capacity or ferritin	
Liver function tests	?Cholestasis
Autoimmune profile	?Antimitochondrial antibodies
Thyroid function tests	?Hyper/hypothyroidism
Urea and electrolytes, creatinine	
Follicle-stimulating hormone, luteinizing hormone (in postmenopausal female)	
?Caeruloplasmin	

measurement of 5-hydroxyindoleacetic acid (5-HIAA) in 24-h urine. Investigation of flushing is well-reviewed by Wilkin (1983).

Atopic dermatitis, urticaria and erythroderma

ATOPIC DERMATITIS (ATOPIC ECZEMA)

Total serum immunoglobulin E (IgE), associated with eosinophilia, is elevated in 80% of patients with atopic dermatitis (atopic eczema), although it is generally not of diagnostic value. Specific IgE antibodies to individual antigens, measured by radioallergoabsorbent test (RAST), correlate reasonably well with positive prick tests. However, routine prick testing is unhelpful; positive reactions are non-specific and may be falsely assumed by the patient to be the cause of the eczema. In practice, a properly controlled exclusion diet is a more effective way of confirming or excluding dietary allergens in atopic dermatitis.

URTICARIA

No routine blood tests are necessary in the average patient with chronic urticaria. A plasma viscosity or erythrocyte sedimentation rate (ESR) may be elevated; a RAST may occasionally confirm a clinical suspicion of a specific antigen. Where there is a history of angioedema, particularly with a positive family history, serum complement C4 and C1 esterase inhibitor should be measured, ideally including a functional assay. Hyperthyroidism may present as symptomatic dermographism. In the patient with chronic unexplained urticaria, a challenge test battery may reveal unsuspected triggers such as salicylates, benzoates, etc.

ERYTHRODERMA

In a red patient with lymphadenopathy, one should check the peripheral blood film for atypical mononuclear cells. Over 10% suggests Sézary syndrome. A lesser percentage is found in other patients with erythroderma. In all patients it is important to monitor renal function.

Problems with hair and nails

DIFFUSE ALOPECIA

In the menstruating female iron deficiency is an important cause of diffuse hair loss. Thyroid function tests may reveal hypothyroidism or, more rarely, hyperthyroidism. An androgenic pattern of hair loss merits measurement of sex hormone-binding globulin and serum testosterone. Where these are abnormal, further investigation is warranted to exclude polycystic ovary disease. Alopecia areata may be associated with other organ-specific autoimmune diseases; an autoimmune profile may show positive thyroid or gastric parietal cell antibodies; it does not affect management. In an infant with sparse, abnormal-looking hair, it is worthwhile screening the urine for inborn errors of metabolism, such as homocystinuria or arginosuccinic aciduria.

EXCESSIVE HAIR GROWTH

The term hirsutism describes excessive hair growth in an androgen-dependent pattern in the female. As this condition merges with normality, endocrine investigations are often normal, in part reflecting different end-organ responses to normal circulating androgens. Hirsutism, associated with acne and oligomenorrhoea, may be a presenting feature of polycystic ovary syndrome; typically the ratio of LH to FSH is increased and testosterone, oestradiol and androstenedione levels are raised. Hirsuties may also be associated with hyperprolactinaemia or, in childhood, with congenital adrenal hyperplasia; the affected child usually has other features of virilization and bizarre electrolyte status due to salt loss. Generalized hypertrichosis (non-androgenic excessive hair growth) may be seen in Cushing's syndrome (idiopathic or iatrogenic), in which plasma cortisol levels will be elevated, and hypothyroidism in children. Hypertrichosis of light-exposed skin occurs in some cases of erythropoietic protoporphyria and almost all of the rarer congenital erythropoietic porphyria (check red-cell porphyrins) and porphyria variegata (check urine porphyrins). It is also seen on the trunk and limbs in mucopolysaccharidoses such as Hurler's syndrome (check urine mucopolysaccharides).

NAIL DISORDERS

Koilonychia is linked with iron deficiency anaemia. One should check thyroid and renal function in patients with yellow-nail syndrome.

Pigmentary disorders

Diffuse pigmentation, especially involving the flexures, suggests Addison's disease (or, paradoxically, sometimes Cushing's syndrome); measure cortisols and, if possible, (β-melanocyte-stimulating hormone β-MSH); a similar pattern is occasionally seen in hyperthyroidism, phaeochromocytoma and carcinoid (check 24-h urine vanillylmandelic acid and 5-HIAA). Numerous asymmetrical, irregular, light-brown macules in a child suggest Albright's syndrome. Bone X-rays, especially of the skull, are of most value, but serum alkaline phosphatase is often elevated.

Yellowish or yellow-brown pigmentation suggests jaundice (check liver function tests) or carotinaemia (check serum carotene levels). Hypermelanosis also occurs in cirrhosis, particularly primary biliary cirrhosis. Greyish pigmentation is a presenting feature of haemochromatosis; blood changes include abnormal liver function tests, raised serum iron and hyperglycaemia. Darkening of the ear cartilage, sclerae and conjunctivae suggests ochronosis (raised urine homogentisic acid). Finally, two rarities: in a boy with brownish pigmentation of the flexures and lower legs, often with depigmented macules, consider Fanconi syndrome (hypoplastic anaemia, thrombocytopenia and neutropenia). Diffuse pigmentation of the neck and extremities, together with alopecia and nail defects, suggests Cronkhite–Canada syndrome (low potassium, calcium and albumin).

Blistering Disorders (Table 3.2)

Disease activity in pemphigus and pemphigoid correlates roughly with the antibodies to intercellular substance and basement membrane respectively. Circulating IgG antibodies, binding to the surface of epithelial cells, are found in almost all patients with pemphigus. However, only 70% of pemphigoid patients exhibit circulating IgG basement membrane zone antibodies, although the detection rate can be increased to 90% using salt-separated skin on indirect immunofluorescence. IgG_1 antibodies are detected in all patients with

---

Table 3.2 Serological investigation of the autoimmune blistering diseases

Disease	Indirect immunofluorescence
Pemphigus vulgaris	Intercellular IgG
Pemphigus foliaceus	
Bullous pemphigoid	IgG/C3, basement membrane (20% IgA)
Herpes (pemphigoid) gestationis	C3, occasional IgG, basement membrane
Linear IgA disease	IgA (children, rare in adults)
Epidermolysis bullosa acquisita	IgG or C3 (dermal on split skin)
Dermatitis herpetiformis	Negative

IgG = Immunoglobulin G.

pemphigoid (herpes) gestationis. Serum gliadin antibodies are found in dermatitis herpetiformis and some cases of pemphigoid; at present it is not a routine procedure. For diagnostic purposes, direct immunofluorescence of perilesional, clinically normal, skin is more rewarding.

Basement membrane antibodies are found in only 25–35% of patients with cicatricial pemphigoid. IgA antibodies are occasionally observed. A circulating IgG autoantibody directed against the upper dermis is found in roughly half of patients with epidermolysis bullosa acquisita. The use of split skin increases the rate of detecting circulating antibodies and enables distinction from bullous pemphigoid.

Indirect immunofluorescence is positive in most children, but few adults, with linear IgA disease. An identical autoantibody is found in bullous systemic lupus erythematosus (SLE). 'Metabolic' bullae occur rarely on the feet and hands in diabetes and in light-exposed areas in renal failure and porphyria cutanea tarda (check urinary porphyrins in a random sample).

Photosensitivity

Congenital and acquired porphyria may present with light sensitivity. Erythropoietic protoporphyria presents typically in childhood. Protoporphyrins are found in the red cells and plasma. Both porphyria cutanea tarda and variegate porphyria are associated with increased uro- and coproporphyrins in the urine. Protoporphyrins dominate in the faeces in porphyria variegata and isocoproporphyrins in porphyria cutanea tarda. Several rarer porphyrinas are described, and if screening tests are negative with a strong clinical likelihood of porphyria, it is worthwhile contacting a reference laboratory.

Photosensitivity is common in lupus erythematosus (LE), especially discoid and subacute forms. Simple screening investigations include antinuclear factor and antibodies to Ro and La (see below).

Purpura and vasculitis

In the patient presenting with purpura, the platelet count may be increased or decreased. In individuals with echymosis or internal bleeding a coagulation screen should include prothrombin time, kaolin cephalin clotting time, thrombin clotting time and fibrinogen. Autoimmune thrombocytopenia may be a presenting feature of SLE; circulating platelet antibodies may be detectable. In the patient with sicca syndrome, purpura on the legs is associated with hypergammaglobulinaemia. Large bruises may be due to defects in collagen, either congenital, as in Ehlers–Danlos syndrome, or acquired, as in scurvy, when plasma vitamin C is decreased.

In cutaneous vasculitis, serological tests are employed, either to determine aetiology, where possible, or to assess the degree of systemic involvement. ESR or viscosity is typically elevated, often greatly so, in giant cell arteritis. Non-specific features of immune complex-mediated damage include the consumption of complement C3 and, to some extent, C4. (However, there may be increased synthesis as part of the acute-phase response.) If possible, it is preferable to measure breakdown fragments such as C3d, C3a and C4a. Measurement of antistreptolysin O titre (ASOT) and anti-DNAase B may elicit a streptococcal cause in patients with Henoch–Schönlein purpura and erythema nodosum. In patients with cutaneous vasculitis a fresh urine sample should be examined on several occasions for protein, red cells and casts. The urine should be re-examined at intervals up to a year after clearance of the cutaneous lesions. Serum creatinine and urea are useful screens; if abnormal, more sophisticated tests of renal function are mandatory.

When vasculitic lesions are precipitated or aggravated by cold, it is worthwhile checking plasma cryoglobulins. A fasting blood sample should be allowed to clot *at 37°C* for 3–4 h. (The serum is then cooled at 4°C for several days.)

Hepatitis B antigen is positive in some patients with polyarteritis nodosa, particularly in the USA.

Some forms of inflammatory panniculitis,

notably with fat liquefaction, are associated with α₁-antitrypsin deficiency. In panniculitis due to pancreatitis or pancreatic carcinoma, serum amylase and urine lipase are typically elevated.

Antineutrophil cytoplasmic antibodies (ANCAs) are found in polymorphs and monocytes. The perinuclear pattern (pANCA) is found non-specifically in vasculitides. Cytoplasmic ANCA is more specific to Wegener's granulomatosis (60–90% of patients).

Vasculitis associated with nodules, especially on extensor surfaces, suggests active rheumatoid disease (rheumatoid factor and antinuclear antibodies (ANA) strongly positive). Urticarial vasculitis is often due to SLE; anti-Sm may be positive (see below).

Cutaneous infarcts may be due to emboli from an atrial myxoma (typically, raised viscosity) or infective endocarditis (check blood cultures).

Connective tissue diseases

Serological tests are often of great value in the differential diagnosis of these patients; in some cases they can offer a guide to prognosis. Non-specific responses to inflammation include a normochromic normocytic anaemia, low serum iron with normal or low iron-binding capacity or transferrin, and an acute-phase response (high ESR or viscosity and raised specific acute-phase proteins, notably C-reactive protein or CRP). However, CRP may be normal or only slightly elevated in SLE. Screening tests should include rheumatoid factor and ANA. Titres of rheumatoid factor and anti-DNA antibodies may be of prognostic significance.

LUPUS ERYTHEMATOSUS

ANA, ideally using Hep-2 cell as a substrate, is nearly always positive in SLE, with lower titres in some patients with discoid and subacute LE (SCLE) (Fig. 3.1). ANA is *not* diagnostic of LE. Double-stranded DNA antibodies are highly specific to SLE, occurring in 70%; they are rare in SCLE and absent in discoid LE. Antibodies to ribonucleoprotein antigens, including Sm (Smith), UI ribonucleoprotein (UIRNP), Ro (SSA) (Fig. 3.2) and La (SSB), are common in SLE. Anti-Sm is specific, found chiefly in Afro-Caribbean and Asiatic patients; it is linked to cutaneous vasculitis. Thirty per cent of SLE patients have antibodies to UIRNP, particularly if there are clinical features of overlap with dermatomyositis or systemic sclerosis; it is usually associated with milder disease and a lower incidence of renal involvement.

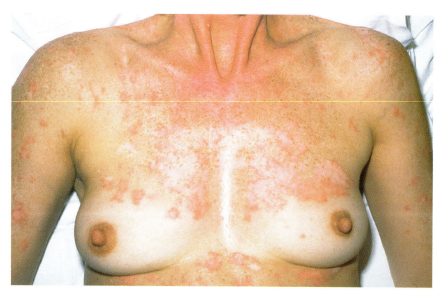

Fig. 3.1 Subacute lupus erythematosus, showing the annular polycyclic configuration of the eruption in a photosensitive distribution.

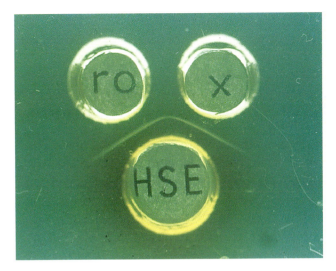

Fig. 3.2 Positive immunodiffusion to Ro in patient's serum (x) with positive control Ro antigen. Courtesy of Prof. P.J. Maddison.

Antibodies to Ro (SSA) and La (SSB) are characteristic of idiopathic Sjögren's syndrome; however, they are present in 30% of patients with SLE. There is a strong association with SCLE (80%) and photosensitivity; in these patients ANA may be negative or weakly positive and direct immunofluorescence of skin may also be negative. Ro and La tend also to be linked to autoimmune purpura and leukopenia. They occur in less than 1% of the normal population. They are strongly associated with neonatal heart block with or without other features of neonatal lupus. The possible pathogenic role of these antibodies is reviewed by Ben-Chetrit (1993). Antibodies to thyroglobulin and thyroid microsomes are found in a third of patients with SLE; 5–10% have clinical thyroid disease.

Anticardiolipin and other antiphospholipid antibodies occur in 20% of SLE patients and are a feature of the related **antiphospholipid syndrome**, including venous and arterial thromboses, strokes, migraine and a history of recurrent spontaneous abortions. They should be measured in patients who present with livedo reticularis and they are linked to false-positive Venereal Disease Reference Laboratory (VDRL) and high levels of IgG. Prothrombin and partial thromboplastin times may be slightly prolonged.

Numerous specific antibodies to clotting factors are found in SLE. It is imperative to check clotting function before embarking on invasive procedures such as renal biopsy.

SCLERODERMA

Anticentromere antibodies are found in 90% of patients with localized forms of systemic sclerosis

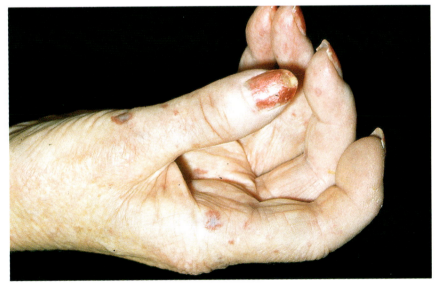

Fig. 3.3 Matt telangiectasia, fingertip atrophy and calcinosis in a patient with CREST syndrome.

(e.g. CREST syndrome; Fig. 3.3) although they are not specific, occurring in some patients with SLE and other connective tissue disorders. In contrast, roughly a third of patients with diffuse scleroderma, bearing a poorer prognosis, exhibit positive antibody titres to Scl-70 (topoisomerase I) Forty per cent of patients with systemic sclerosis possess antibodies to nucleolar components, including RNA polymerase I (associated with myositis). Screening tests of renal function should be repeated regularly, such as 6-monthly. Thermography, if available, is useful to quantify the degree of vasospasm in Raynaud's phenomenon and to monitor the effect of drugs. Nailfold capillaroscopy typically shows avascular areas and dilated, irregular capillaries in diffuse systemic sclerosis.

Radiological investigation, including barium swallow and small-bowel follow-through, is useful to determine the degree of gastrointestinal involvement. Other important investigations include the single-breath diffusion test, which is abnormal in over 70% of patients with diffuse disease, computed tomographic scans of the lungs, electrocardiogram and echocardiograph, and joint X-rays.

Remember that scleroderma-like changes in the hands are seen in insulin-dependent diabetes mellitus.

Patients with localized morphoea frequently have positive organ-specific autoantibodies on routine screening. Diffuse morphoea with panniculitis is often associated with blood eosinophilia and may be confused with eosinophilic fasciitis.

DERMATOMYOSITIS (Fig. 3.4)

Serum creatinine (phospho) kinase (CK) is the most useful measure of muscle damage; the isoenzyme CK-MM is most specific for skeletal muscle. Some laboratories measure serum aldolase and urinary creatine/creatinine ratio. Non-specific features in dermatomyositis include a positive ANA in 40%.

Antibodies to Jo-I (histidyl t-RNA synthetase) occur in 20% of patients with polymyositis, especially with interstitial lung disease. These antibodies occur occasionally in dermatomyositis, and may be linked with 'mechanic's hands' (psoriasiform lesions on the hands). Other synthetase antibodies may also have specific disease associations, for example, Mi-2 with more typical dermatomyositis. Electromyography (EMG) of affected muscles characteristically shows spontaneous fibrillation and polyphasic myopathic potentials. Muscle biopsy, if required, should be carried out on clinically abnormal muscle, on the opposite side, thus avoiding histological EMG changes.

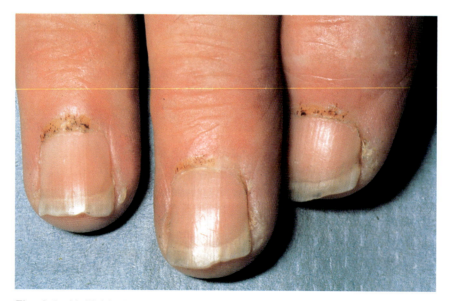

Fig. 3.4 Nailfold telangiectasia in dermatomyositis.

Magnetic resonance imaging (MRI) can detect areas of inflammatory myopathy.

Infections

VIRAL

Although a diagnosis can sometimes be achieved by a single high antibody titre, it is usually preferable to examine paired sera, the first taken as soon as possible after onset of symptoms and the second after 10 days (5–7 days in rubella). A four-fold rise in titre is generally diagnostic.

Infectious mononucleosis may present as urticaria, a morbilliform eruption (characteristically induced by ampicillin) or occasionally with genital ulceration. A blood film reveals lymphocytosis with some cellular atypia. Liver function tests are often abnormal. The diagnosis is usually confirmed by the Paul-Bunnell test (heterophile antibodies which agglutinate sheep or horse red cells). In acute HIV infection, the virus can sometimes be cultured from peripheral lymphocytes. Seroconversion may take 1–6 months. Electron microscopy of blister fluid can be positive in an early herpes simplex vesicle. The Tzanck smear is also useful (Chapter 2).

BACTERIAL

β-Haemolytic streptococci are recognized triggers of guttate psoriasis and cutaneous vasculitis, including erythema nodosum. In early stages, streptococci may be isolated on a throat swab. The ASOT and, more specifically, the anti-DNAase B, may be raised in serum. Blood cultures (ideally three separate samples) may demonstrate bacteraemia in infective endocarditis, meningococcal meningitis or gonococcal infections. Brucellosis can occasionally be diagnosed by blood culture, although a raised titre of specific agglutinins is more useful (a titre over 1:300 is diagnostic: 1:100–300 is suspicious).

In erythema chronicum migrans or Lyme disease, *Borrelia burgdorferi* titres become positive within a few weeks of infection. Serological tests for syphilis include reagin tests, the most common used being flocculation tests (e.g. VDRL); these are helpful in screening and assessing disease activity. Biological false-positive reactions occur in connective tissue diseases. A specific treponemal antibody test (e.g. *Treponema pallidum* haemagglutination test) is essential to establish a diagnosis; however, false-positive reactions also occur in other spirochaete infections (e.g. Lyme disease, yaws).

In a patient presenting with erythema multiforme and respiratory symptoms, it is worth checking antibodies to *Mycoplasma pneumoniae*. Specific antibody titres are available for the diagnosis of more exotic rickettsiae and chlamydiae. Circulating antibodies to *Mycobacterium leprae* are found in most patients with lepromatous leprosy.

FUNGI/YEASTS

Persistent candidal infection of skin, mouth and nails may reflect a primary immune defect, e.g. Swiss-type agammaglobulinaemia. It may also be linked with a polyendocrinopathy (hypothyroidism or hypoparathyroidism with Addison's disease).

Serological tests are useful in diagnosing systemic fungal infections such as cryptococcosis or histoplasmosis.

PROTOZOA

Trypanosomiasis can be diagnosed by thin blood films, as for malaria, or serology. Serum *Leishmania* antibodies can be demonstrated in patients with visceral leishmaniasis.

Metabolic disorders

LIPID ABNORMALITIES

Widespread lipoatrophy in the adult may reflect hyperlipidaemia or an endocrine abnormality such as elevated growth hormone or hyperthyroidism. High titres of thyroid antibodies are found in many patients with partial lipoatrophy. More importantly, hypocomplementaemia (low C3, normal C4) in these patients is strongly associated with circulating C3 'nephritic' factor and glomerulonephritis.

Serum lipids may be raised in patients with gout, xanthomata, xanthelasma palpebrarum and multicentric reticulohistiocytosis. In this last condition, X-rays of the hands show a severe erosive arthritis of the distal interphalangeal joints.

MUCOPOLYSACCHARIDE ABNORMALITIES

Pretibial myxoedema is strongly linked with hyperthyroidism. Serum IgG paraprotein is found by electrophoresis in some patients with lichen myxoedematosus. Urine mucopolysaccharides are elevated in childhood disorders such as Hunter's and Hurler's syndromes.

AMYLOIDOSIS

Histology is essential for accurate diagnosis. In nodular cutaneous amyloidosis the ESR and β and γ– globulins may be raised. Urine positive for Bence Jones protein suggests associated myeloma in systemic amyloidosis. If a plasma cell dyscrasia is suspected, immunoelectrophoresis of serum and concentrated urine is the most sensitive technique for detecting monoclonal paraprotein.

DISORDERS OF AMINO ACID METABOLISM

- Phenylketonuria: raised plasma phenylalanine, raised urine phenylpyruvic acid (may be normal in the first few months).
- Richner–Hanhart syndrome: raised plasma and urine tyrosine.
- Alkaptonuria: raised urine homogentisic acid – looks dark.
- Homocystinuria: raised urine homocystine.
- Hartnup disease: raised urine indican.

VITAMIN DISORDERS

Patients with beri-beri excrete less than 50 μg of aneurin in 24 h urine after ingestion of 1 mg.

In scurvy, serum vitamin C is decreased (normal range 17–94 μmol/L).

ICHTHYOSES

The precise biochemical diagnosis is chiefly made in research laboratories by analysis of scale or fibroblast cultures. In Refsum's syndrome, high blood levels of phytanic acid are found (992–6400 μmol/L), the normal range being 0–33 μmol/L.

Acanthosis nigricans, especially presenting before puberty, can be associated with a variety of endocrine disorders, including hyperandrogenism and insulin resistance.

MISCELLANEOUS

Anderson–Fabry disease (angiokeratoma corporis diffusum): α-galactosidase is decreased in plasma and leukocytes; birefringent lipid-containing cells are seen in the urine.

In gout, check serum uric acid, lipids and monitor renal function. An erosive arthritis may be demonstrated on X-rays of the affected joints. Serum zinc is decreased (normal range 70–125 μmol/ml) in acrodermatitis enteropathica and acquired zinc deficiency.

Other inflammatory disorders

In acute sarcoidosis, the ESR is raised within 6–8 weeks of onset of erythema nodosum, and may be linked with lung involvement. A chest X-ray may show bilateral hilar lymphadenopathy. There is often hypercalcaemia and hypercalciuria. The angiotensin-converting enzyme is not specific but it is useful to monitor disease activity. In chronic sarcoidosis, X-rays of the hands and feet may reveal cystic changes in the phalanges (sarcoid dactylitis) and the chest X-ray may show pulmonary fibrosis. A gallium scan will reveal areas of disease activity.

Plasma glucagon is raised in necrotic migratory erythema.

A neutrophilia is typical of Sweet's syndrome; this disorder and pyoderma gangrenosum may be presenting features of leukaemia or paraproteinaemia.

Remember to check HIV status in patients with Reiter's syndrome (after appropriate counselling).

MONITORING DRUGS COMMONLY USED IN DERMATOLOGY

Table 3.3 Monitoring drugs commonly used in dermatology

Drug	Baseline assessment	During therapy
Acyclovir (intravenous)	Urea, creatinine	Urea, creatinine
Azathioprine*	FBC, LFTs	FBC, LFTs (1–2 weeks, then bimonthly)
Calcipotriol (topical)	Calcium (corrected)	Calcium (corrected) if usage greater then 100g/week, less if psoriasis unstable
Colchicine	FBC, U&E, creatinine	FBC, U&E, creatinine
Cyclosporin	Serum creatinine (at least × 2) Assess GFR ?plus renal plasma flow	Creatinine. U&E (2-weekly for 2–3 months then monthly). Repeat GFR after long-term use
Dapsone	FBC, differential and platelets. G6PD level, if appropriate, LFTs, U&E	FBC, differential WCC and reticulocytes (2-weekly for 3 months, then 2–3-monthly), U&E, LFTs
Hydroxyurea	FBC and platelets LFTS, urea, creatinine, uric acid	FBC and platelets weekly for 1–2 months, then monthly. Other tests 3–6-monthly
Methotrexate	FBC and differential WCC, LFTS	FBC and differential WCC and platelets. LFTs (only detect hepatocellular toxicity) 1–2-weekly for 3 months then 1–2-monthly. NB: Currently no adequate substitute for liver biopsy, although serum level of amino-terminal type III procollagen peptide looks promising
PUVA	LFTs, ANA and extractable nuclear antigen (ENA)	
Aromatic retinoids	Fasting lipids, LFTs	Fasting lipids, LFTS after 4–6 weeks, then 1–2-monthly (in high-risk patients check lipids after 2 weeks)

FBC = Full blood count; LFTs = liver function tests; U&E = urea and electrolytes; GFR = glomenrular filtration rate; G6PD = glucose-6-phosphate dehydrogenase; WCC, white cell count; ANA, antinuclear antibody

* It seems that about 1 in 300 patients receiving azathioprine are at risk of life-threatening myelosuppression, due to low or absent levels of thiopurine methyltransferase (TPMT) activity, with resultant metabolism to 6-thioguanine nucleotides (6-TGN). In order to predict these patients, assays for either TPMT itself or 6-TGN levels are presently being developed for routine use.

FURTHER READING

Archer CB. Atopic dermatitis – an obvious diagnosis? *Clinical and Experimental Dermatology* 1986; **11**: 560–563.

Ben-Chetrit E. The molecular basis of the SSA/Ro antigens and the clinical significance of their autoantibodies. *British Journal of Rheumatology* 1993; **32**: 396–402.

Chan H–L, Lee Y–S, Hong HS, Kuo T–T. Anticentromere antibodies (ACA): clinical distribution and disease specificity. *Clinical and Experimental Dermatology* 1994; **19**: 298–302.

Conway GS, Honour JW, Jacobs HS. Heterogeneity of the polycystic ovary syndrome: clinical, endocrine and ultrasound features in 536 patients. *Clinical Endocrinology* 1989; **30**: 459–464.

Denman ST. A review of pruritus. *Journal of the American Academy of Dermatology* 1986; **14**: 375–392.

Kallenberg CGM. Antineutrophil cytoplasmic antibodies (ANCA) and vasculitis. *Clinical Rheumatology* 1990; **9**: 132–35.

Kirtschig G, Wojnarowska H. Autoimmune blistering disease: an update of diagnostic methods and investigations. *Clinical and Experimental Dermatology* 1994; **19**: 97–112.

Lennard L, Van Loon JA, Weinshilboum RM. Pharmacogenetics of acute azathioprine toxicity: relationship to thiopurine methyltransferase genetic polmorphism. *Clinical Pharmacoology and Therapeutics* 1989; **46**: 149–154.

Lovell CR, Maddison PJ, Campion GV. *The Skin in Rheumatic Disease*. Chapman & Hall Medical, London, 1990.

Wilkin JK. Flushing reactions. In: Rook AJ, Maibach HI (eds) *Recent Advances in Dermatology*, no. 6. Churchill Livingstone, Edinburgh, 1983, pp. 157–187.

Wolverton S. Monitoring for adverse effects from systemic drugs used in dermatology. *Journal of the American Academy of Dermatology* 1992; **26**: 661–679.

Chapter 4

Investigation of allergic skin disorders and the photodermatoses

Gillian M. Murphy

Allergic skin disorders are caused by antigens in contact with the skin or mucous membranes, or present systemically. Once sensitization has occurred, further contact with the allergen leads to reproducible reactions. Skin diseases with an allergic basis are common and categorized into those caused by immediate or delayed type hypersensitivity. Immediate reactions (type I) are immunoglobulin E (IgE)-mediated. Delayed reactions may be IgG or IgM antibody (type II), immune complex (type III) or T-cell (type IV)-mediated. Table 4.1 lists examples of immediate and delayed reactions.

Irritant reactions (e.g. nettle sting) are much commoner than allergic urticarial reactions such as hypersensitivity to ingested foods or immediate contact hypersensitivity (Table 4.2). Delayed cell-mediated reactions are caused by commonly encountered allergens, for example, allergic contact dermatitis caused by nickel, or occupationally encountered allergens, such as rubber or cement. Allergic contact dermatitis accounts for 30% of occupationally associated skin diseases. Irritant contact dermatitis is even commoner, being relevant in 60% of occupational dermatitis.

Allergic reactions may be complex, particularly in patients with endogenous eczema and photosensitivity. Clinical examination and history may not distinguish between constitutional eczema, allergic and irritant reactions. Unfortunately, many patients have a mixed picture of endogenous eczema complicated by either allergic or irritant contact dermatitis, or both. All contributing causes therefore must be addressed. Identification of IgE-mediated reactions to allergens such as the house dust mite or animal dander is frequent in atopic dermatitis (atopic eczema), but dust avoidance may not improve the patient. The art of good management of patients with eczema is the ability to determine in an individual patient which factors are most relevant to the exacerbation or perpetuation of disease. This depends on a good clinical history combined with appropriate investigations.

Table 4.1 Examples of immediate and delayed hypersensitivity

Immediate hypersensitivity	Delayed hypersensitivity
Contact urticaria	Contact dermatitis
Solar urticaria	Photocontact dermatitis
Drug-induced urticaria	Drug-induced dermatitis
Food-induced urticaria	Food-induced dermatitis
	Vasculitis
	Erythema multiforme
	Thrombocytopenic purpura

Table 4.2 Allergic contact urticaria

Animal dander, saliva, serum

Plant products: wood, strawberries, rubber

Foods: eggs, flour, fruit, vegetables, meat

Cosmetics: hair and nail products, perfume

Medicaments: antibiotics

Textiles: silk, wool, nylon

TESTS OF IMMEDIATE HYPERSENSITIVITY

Skin tests

The technique involves application of a minute quantity of allergen to the skin, and for a **prick test**, insertion of a sterile stylet or needle at 45° to breach the epidermis, enabling penetration of the allergen, without drawing blood (bleeding leads to false-positive reactions). After 15 min the allergens are removed, test sites inspected, and the diameter of induced wheals measured and graded in comparison to a positive and negative control. Histamine 1 and 10 mg/ml is used as a positive control. Glycerol 50% in aqueous solution, the vehicle for the allergen solutions, is a negative control. Standard series of allergens containing the commonest antigens, such as house dustmite, pollen, dairy produce, nuts, fish and wheat, are commercially available (Dome Hollister-Stier, USA).

Intradermal injection of allergen and **scratch tests** are potentially more dangerous, with a risk of anaphylaxis in very susceptible subjects (for example, in peanut allergy). Prick testing plays a limited role in the management of patients now that desensitization of patients with hay fever and asthma is rarely undertaken, due to the risk of anaphylactic shock. Multiple positive reactions are indicative of atopy, but the reactions must be carefully interpreted as they may be clinically irrelevant. Immediate reactions may be followed by a late-phase reaction, which may explain why immediate hypersensitivity is relevant in patients with hand dermatitis. In caterers, for example, positive prick tests to foods (Fig. 4.1) document contact urticaria and explain the itching and burning which such patients describe after handling some foods. The use of control subjects allows irritant reactions to be distinguished from allergic reactions. Avoidance of implicated foods

may lead to clinical improvement. Prick tests may not be used reliably to diagnose systemic food allergy in atopic dermatitis, as both false-positive and negative results commonly occur.

IgE and radioallergoabsorbent tests (RASTs)

Serum IgE measurement is a routine clinical test: 1 IU = 2.4 ng/ml IgE. If IgE exceeds the normal range – usually > 100 IU – it is indicative of atopy; however, a normal IgE does not rule out atopy. RASTs (Fig. 4.2) which measure antigen-specific IgE are commercially available, variable in specificity and, like prick tests, are of limited value. A positive RAST does not indicate causality. Patients may have high levels of reactivity against house-dust mite, but be in clinical remission. A negative RAST does not rule out allergy; it merely indicates that the allergen tested did not detect antibody, either because an inappropriate antigen was used or, at the time of testing, the patient was not producing antibody against the allergen.

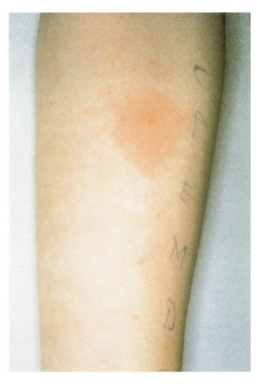

Fig. 4.1 Positive prick test to foods (in caterers)

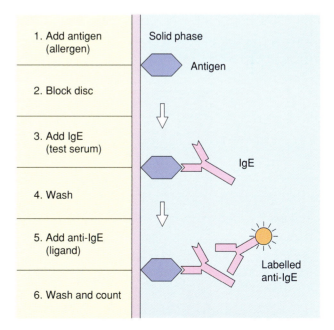

Fig. 4.2 The radioallergoabsorbent test (RAST) measuring antigen-specific immunoglobulin E (IgE) in a radioimmunoassay where the ligand is a labelled anti-IgE antibody.

Food allergy in atopic dermatitis

The only reliable method of documenting true food allergy as an exacerbating factor in atopic dermatitis is by instituting a strict allergen-free diet followed by double-blind challenge of excluded foods. Intradermal tests and RASTs are not reliable markers of food allergy in atopic dermatitis. Most commonly, dairy products are suspected. The patient takes a dairy produce-free diet for a defined period of time (usually 6–8 weeks). If there is no improvement, dairy products are deemed irrelevant.

Clinical improvement during this time may reflect the natural history of atopic dermatitis, which fluctuates in severity, or the effects of treatment. It is therefore important to show that ingestion of the food causes worsening of the eczema after a period of dietary restriction.

There are many reasons why foods induce reactions in infants which are misconstrued as allergies. Perhaps commonest is food ingestion leading to increased body temperature; this causes facial erythema and itch, leading to scratching, particularly in those with severe eczema. Inappropriately restrictive diets in a child with eczema compound the difficulties of the child and parents, so careful analysis of the need for the diet is advisable.

PATCH TESTING

Patch testing is a standardized method of distinguishing allergic from irritant contact dermatitis. It is extremely useful in determining the cause of allergic contact dermatitis and can result in cure when a causative allergen is avoided. Patch testing does not diagnose irritant contact dermatitis. Patch testing is fraught with difficulties, and in inexperienced hands incorrect interpretation of reactions is common. False-positive and false-negative reactions are common and ways of minimizing these reactions must be employed. Test procedures are usually carried out by a trained nurse, and readings performed by an experienced dermatologist.

Patch tests are carried out using aluminium Finn chambers, usually 8 mm in diameter, mounted on non-allergic adhesive tape (Fig. 4.3). These are commercially available as 10 chambers per strip; the distance between chambers is optimized to separate individual reactions. The upper back is the preferred site for testing (Fig. 4.4), enabling as many as 50–100 allergens to be tested. The position of the individual chambers must be clearly marked to identify reactions, using a non-allergenic waterproof skin-marking pen, or tape. Tape adheres poorly in patients with very dry skin; the marker pen may be erased with oily

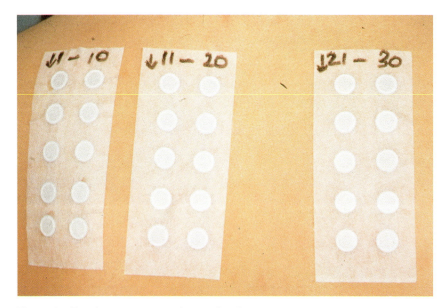

Fig. 4.3 Patch tests mounted on adhesive tape.

sweating skin. Poor results accrue from poor compliance, therefore written instructions to patients are helpful.

The commonest sensitizing agents have been identified and agreed by the International Contact Dermatitis Research Group. The European Standard Series (Table 4.3) is updated periodically in line with the most frequent occurring sensitizers. These tests identify 70% of cases of allergic contact dermatitis. Additional batteries appropriate to many different occupations and clinical situations (facial, hairdressers, nurses, medicaments, etc.) greatly improve sensitivity and accuracy. A careful history should be taken and a clinical examination performed in each patient to decide whether allergens apart from the Standard Series should be applied. Patch-testing centres may add allergens appropriate to the local population to the Standard Series. In my practice, a steroid series (Tables 4.4 and 4.5) is added to the standard series, with positive findings in 3% of patients tested. These steroid-sensitive patients would otherwise be missed.

The order in which allergens are applied is important as some allergens give irritant or vigorous allergic reactions. To avoid false-positives, such allergens are best spaced out. Vehicles used for allergen delivery are relatively inert:

petrolatum, water, methylethylketone and alcohol. Cosmetics are applied neat or, if strong reactions are anticipated, diluted. Great care must be employed when testing unknown chemicals as severe chemical burns with skin necrosis may result. Acids and alkalis should be avoided; if in doubt, the agent may be diluted and used as an open test initially. Liquids are applied on filter paper discs within Finn chambers. Solid substances are reduced to dust, fabrics moistened and applied in the chamber. Pressure from hard fragments may lead to false positives; false negatives may arise from low allergen concentration.

The method and timing of readings are most important. Patch tests are removed after 48h, the first reading is performed, documented, and 2 days later a further reading is carried out. The skin may appear inflamed immediately after removal of the strips, or pressure from the chamber may blanch a positive test, and readings are best carried out 20–30 min later. Tests should be read in bright daylight or with fluorescent lighting. Some allergens penetrate the skin slowly, and there may not be any reactions at the first reading, but by the second reading, the reaction is evident. Reactions may appear later than this, so patients should watch for delayed reactions and return for assessment if possible. Table 4.6 shows

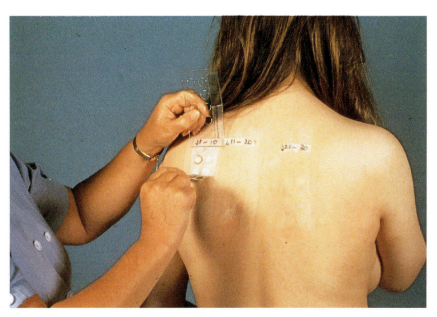

Fig. 4.4 Patch testing on the upper back.

Table 4.3 The standard European patch-testing series

Substance	Concentration
Potassium dichromate	0.5%
Neomycin sulphate	20.0%
Thiuram mix	1.0%
Paraphenylenediamine (PPD)	1.0%
Cobalt chloride	1.0%
Benzocaine	5.0%
Formaldehyde	1.0%
Colophony	20.0%
Clioquinol	5.0%
Balsam of Peru	25.0%
Isopropyl-phenyl-*p*-phenylenediamine	0.1%
Wool alcohols	30.0%
Mercapto mix	2.0%
Epoxy resin	1.0%
Paraben mix	15.0%
Paratertiarybutyl phenol formaldehyde resin	1.0%
Fragrance mix	8.0%
Quaternium 15 (Dowicil)	1.0%
Nickel sulphate	5.0%
Isothiazoline mix	0.01%
Mercaptobenzothiazole	2.0%
Sesquitertpene lactone mix	0.1%
Primin	0.01%

Table 4.4 Allergens commonly added to Standard Series

Ethylenediamine*	1.0%
Tixocortol pivalate	1.0%
Budesonide	0.1%
Triamcinolone acetonide	0.1%
Hydrocortisone 17 butyrate	0.1%
Betamethasone valerate	0.12%
Clobetasol-17-propionate	0.25%
Hydrocortisone	1.0%
Prednisolone	1.0%
Amcinonide	0.1%

* Ethylenediamine formerly in the standard series is found in some steroid-containing creams (Kenacomb and Tri-Adcortyl).

Table 4.5 Face series

Hydrogenated lanolin

Eucerin

Santolite resin

Phosphorus sesquisulphide

Butylated hydroxyanisole

Tertiary butylated hydroxytoluine

Imidazolidinyl urea (Germall 115)

Diazolidinyl urea (Germall II)

Chloracetamide

Bronopol

grading of patch-test reactions. Sources of patch-test material are listed in Table 4.7.

Figure 4.5 shows a classical allergic reaction to the patient's own perfume, with non-specific reactions at other test sites which had faded at the time of the second reading. Irritant reactions may be difficult to interpret; knowing which allergens tend to give irritant reactions is helpful. Nickel is one of the most frequent offenders. Others include cobalt chloride and chromate. These three (the so-called 'atopic triad') may be seen as irritant reactions in patients with atopic dermatitis. Features of an irritant reaction include pustules,

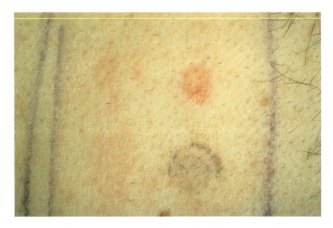

Fig. 4.6 Pustules; sharp ring-like irritant reactions.

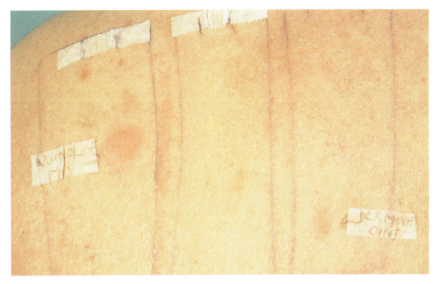

Fig. 4.5 Typical allergic reaction to quinoline mix and dermovate.

an edge effect where there is a sharp ring-like reaction (Fig. 4.6), rapid fading of the reaction after removal of the Finn chambers so that the reaction is fading, often with desquamation at the time of the second reading. Allergic reactions

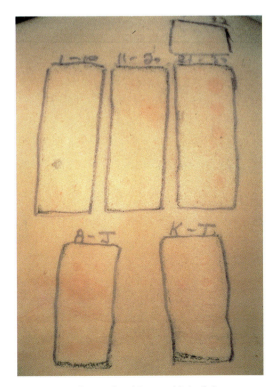

Fig. 4.7 'Angry back' – multiple false-positives and perfume allergy.

Table 4.6	Grading of patch test reactions*
–	Negative
±	Doubtful (feint erythema)
+	Weak (definite erythema)
++	Strong (oedema/vesicles)
+++	Extreme (bullous/erosion)
NT	Not tested
IR	Irritant reaction

* Although grading of patch test reactions is useful, it is difficult to interpret the relative importance of weak, strong or extreme positive reactions, and one should probably decide simply between a positive or negative reaction.

Table 4.7	Commercially available patch-test material

Hermal Kurt Herrmann, PO Box 1228, D-21462 Reinbek/Hamburg, Germany

Chemotechnique Diagnostics AB Ringuggnsgatan 7, S-21616 Malmo, Sweden

Pharmacia Diagnostics S-75182 Uppsala, Sweden

American Academy of Dermatology 1567 Maple Ave, Evanston, Il 60201 USA

have a crescendo pattern, becoming better defined by the second reading. The so-called **'angry back'** is an important source of error, where multiple false positives develop (Fig. 4.7) in the vicinity of a strong reaction from one allergen or if the patient has active eczema at the time of patch testing. More than four reactions should make one suspect an angry back. The offending allergen is later omitted to permit retesting.

Reapplication of an allergen is helpful if the reaction is doubtful at the first reading. Irritant reactions may not recur and allergic reactions are reproducible. If the reaction is florid at the first reading, dilution by 1 in 2 or 1 in 4 will reduce irritancy and enable demonstration of an allergic reaction, when a dose–response effect may be seen. If the reaction is feint, as happens from time to time when testing a cosmetic, but seems clinically relevant, repeat testing using a larger Finn chamber of 16 mm diameter may confirm allergy without increasing the concentration.

A **usage test** (**open test**) is a very helpful adjunct to patch testing. The patient applies the agent twice daily to the skin inferior to the antecubital fossa and production of eczema indicates the relevance of the agent. The production of no reaction after 3 days indicates a false-positive patch test.

Photopatch testing

Interaction of ultraviolet (UV) radiation with some compounds causes an allergenic photoproduct leading to photocontact dermatitis. Application of the allergen alone in the absence of UV radiation leads to no reaction. Modification of the patch-testing technique enables diagnosis of these reactions. There is as yet no standard photoallergen series. The current literature suggests that sunscreens are the commonest photoallergens, and other compounds previously deemed important now seem to be rare. Table 4.8 lists a photoallergen series. These are applied in duplicate for 48 h, removed and read. One set is recovered with opaque material and the other is irradiated with 0.5 J/cm² UVA using a broad-band

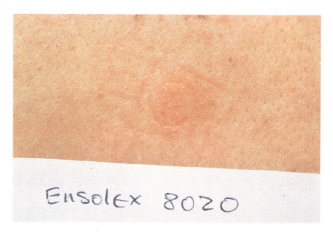

Ensolex 8020

Fig. 4.8 Reactions occurring at ultraviolet-irradiated site deemed positive.

source (measured by an appropriate UVA meter) and re-covered. The tests are read again after 48 h at the time of the second reading of the patch tests. Reactions occurring at the UV-irradiated site are deemed positive (Fig. 4.8). If the non-irradiated tests also react, the reaction is a contact dermatitis.

Care must be taken to exclude phototoxic reactions which are common, particularly with drugs

Table 4.8 Photopatch series	
Chlorpromazine	0.1%
Promethazine	0.1%
Musk ambrette	5.0%
Para-aminobenzoic acid	10.0%
2-Ethylhexyl-p-dimethylamino-benzoate	10.0%
Mexonone	10.0%
Ethoxyethyl-p-methoxy cinnamate	10.0%
1-4-isopropylphenyl-3-phenyl-3-propanedione	10.0%
4-Tert-butyl-4-methoxy-dibenzoylmethane	10.0%
2-Ethyl hexyl-p-methoxy cinnamate	10.0%
Oxybenzone	10.0%
3-4-Methylbenzylidene camphor	10.0%

such as promethazine and chlorpromazine and topical non-steroidal anti-inflammatory agents. Higher UV dosage leads to more frequent phototoxic reactions. Most photoallergic reactions are detected with doses of 1–2 J/cm² UVA, 5 J/cm² UVA is now the agreed European Standard. Patients who are photosensitive should first have an assessment of UV sensitivity and if the **minimal erythema dose** (MED) is found to be less than 5 J/cm², should be tested at 70% of the measured MED. Careful photopatch testing is rewarding in many patients with photodermatoses in whom sunscreen allergy is now the commonest photoallergic reaction seen.

Who should be patch tested?

Twenty per cent of patients with endogenous eczema when patch-tested have a relevant positive patch test. Any patient with eczema, whether atopic, seborrhoeic, palmoplantar, venous or of other evident cause, but where management proves difficult, should be patch-tested as medica-

ments – even topical steroids – may be implicated. All patients with a history and clinical picture suggestive of contact dermatitis should also be tested, even if an allergic cause appears evident; patients with a friction dermatitis from a heavy watch may be inappropriately labelled as having nickel dermatitis. Patients with facial eczema should be tested to the standard series and also to the facial, and if indicated to a cosmetic and photopatch series. All patients with a history suggestive of chronic actinic dermatitis should have patch and photopatch tests. Patients with polymorphic light eruption may likewise benefit as perfume and sunscreen allergies are not uncommon in this group of patients.

INVESTIGATION OF PHOTOSENSITIVE DISEASES

Photosensitivity is very common. Present evidence suggests that some of the idiopathic photodermatoses are allergic in origin; UV radiation induces a delayed hypersensitivity reaction.

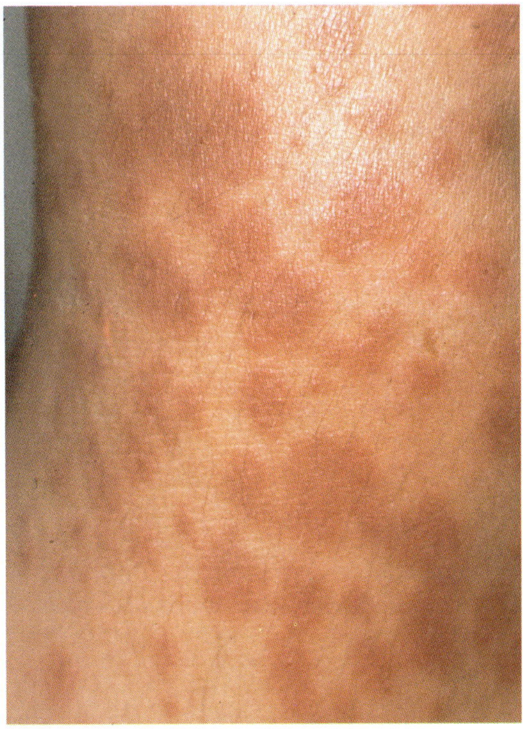

Fig. 4.9 Polymorphic light eruption (PLE).

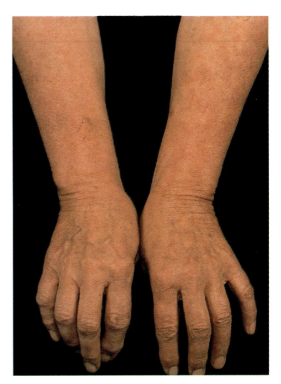

Fig. 4.10 Exclusion of lupus erythematosus, subacute variety.

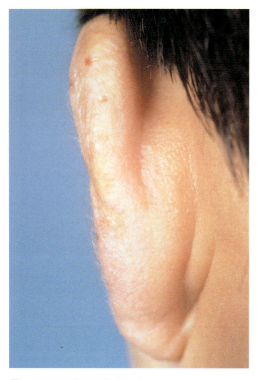

Fig. 4.11 Juvenile spring eruption.

The nature of the allergen is unknown. Polymorphic light eruption (PLE; Fig. 4.9) affects 10–15% of the population. Investigation of PLE includes exclusion of lupus erythematosus, particularly the subacute variety (Fig. 4.10), by testing antinuclear, extractable nuclear antibodies (Ro and La) and by a skin biopsy for histology and direct immunofluorescence if lesions are present. The rash of lupus is usually more severe and longer-lasting compared with that of PLE. Photoallergic contact dermatitis may need to be excluded by patch and photopatch testing, as patients with PLE and other types of photosensitivity may also develop sunscreen allergy as a consequence of frequent use of sunscreens.

Juvenile spring eruption (Fig. 4.11) seems to be a mild transient form of PLE localized to the outer helix of the ears, most frequently seen in boys. Tolerance to the sun usually develops with continued exposure, and further investigation is usually not necessary.

Actinic prurigo (AP) (Fig. 4.12) is an itchy photosensitivity disorder in children, occasionally

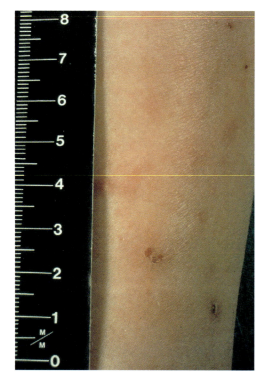

Fig. 4.12 Actinic prurigo.

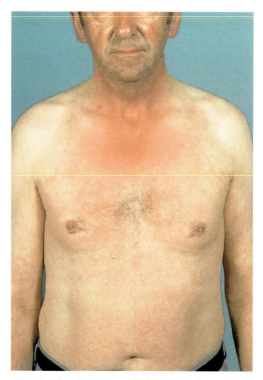

Fig. 4.13 Chronic actinic dermatitis

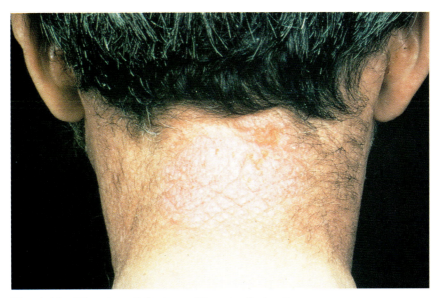

Fig. 4.14 Chronic actinic dermatitis cut-off at collar.

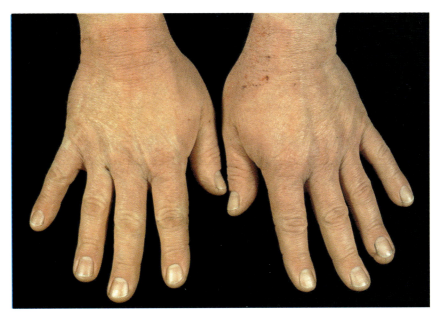

Fig. 4.15 Chronic actinic dermatitis cut-off at cuffs.

persisting or beginning in adult life. Excoriated lesions affect UV-exposed sites, sparing covered areas, but may occur on the lower back and buttocks. Most patients have HLA D4 0407.

Chronic actinic dermatitis (CAD, Fig. 4.13) is a severe photosensitive eczema which predominantly affects elderly men; the prevalence is approximately 1/100000. Patients may not notice that sun exposure exacerbates the rash. Severe lichenified eczema affects the face, back of the neck, V of the chest and backs of the hands. A sharp cut-off is noted at the collar line (Fig. 4.14) and the cuffs (Fig. 4.15). Light-shielded areas under the chin and behind the ears are spared. If the patient becomes erythrodermic, these signs are obscured. CAD is included in the differential diagnosis of erythroderma and air-borne contact dermatitis. Certain types of porphyria may present with a light-induced eruption (Chapter 3).

Assessment of photosensitivity

Patients with photosensitivity are investigated depending on the type of photosensitivity, and on the mode of presentation. All patients thought to have CAD should have the diagnosis confirmed by monochromator testing (see below). The diagnosis of CAD may not be made in the absence of abnormal responses to UV radiation. Patients with CAD should also have patch and photopatch testing, as these patients have a tendency to have multiple allergies, in particular, reactions to fragrance, colophony, sunscreens and the daisy-like group of plants, the Compositae.

PLE patients may need no more than exclusion of lupus erythematosus if the rash is present and typical of PLE at the time of review. Many patients are seen at a time when the rash is not present and it may then be useful to induce the rash to document photosensitivity.

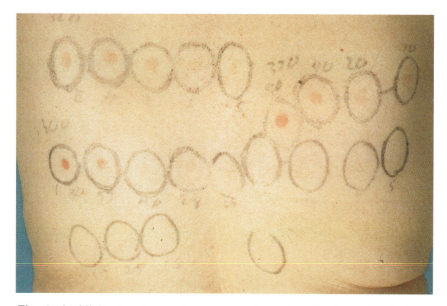

Fig. 4.16 Minimal erythema dose range of wavelengths throughout ultraviolet A and B and visible light.

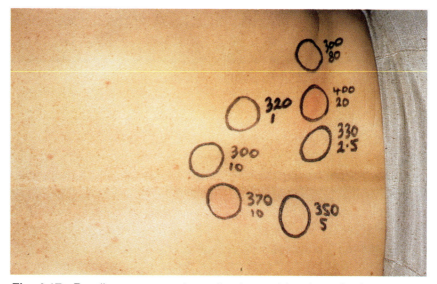

Fig. 4.17 Reading responses immediately as with solar urticaria.

MONOCHROMATOR TESTS

A monochromator is a UV-emitting device which enables testing of patients to individual wavebands of UV radiation and visible light. A high intensity lamp source, usually a xenon arc, emits broad-spectrum UV and visible light, together with infrared radiation. By means of a diffraction grating which breaks the UV into its component wavelengths, a series of focusing mirrors, lenses and appropriate filters, it is possible to produce pure UV of individual wavelengths, within narrow wavebands, as chosen by the clinician. The patient's MED, the dose which produces just perceptible confluent definite erythema for a range of chosen wavelengths throughout the UVB (290–315 nm), UVA (315–400 nm) and visible light range, is documented, at 24 h (Fig. 4.16). It may be appropriate to read responses immediately as with solar urticaria (Fig. 4.17), or at 72 h as with xeroderma pigmentosum, where delayed abnormal erythema responses are characteristic.

Monochromator irradiation tests (MITs)

enable documentation of wavelengths which induce the patient's skin disease, the so-called action spectrum. These tests are most useful in CAD where they are nearly always positive, unless the patient has only recently developed photosensitivity, in which case they may be at first normal. Repeat testing 12 months later enables confirmation or exclusion of the diagnosis of CAD.

Other disorders in which MITs are useful include solar urticaria, where the action spectrum again is determined and the nature of the disorder is evident as the tests induce urticarial wheals on the skin. Seventy per cent of patients with PLE and actinic prurigo have normal responses to MIT; patients with severe disease tend to have abnormal responses. Where photosensitivity is clinically suspected, as in drug-induced photosensitivity and miscellaneous disorders, including lupus erythematosus and in rare disorders such as trichothiodystrophy, MITs may also be helpful confirmatory tests.

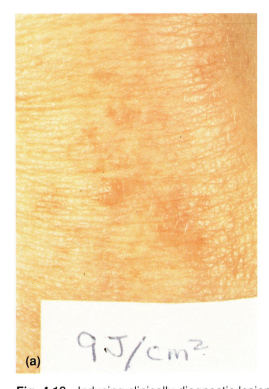 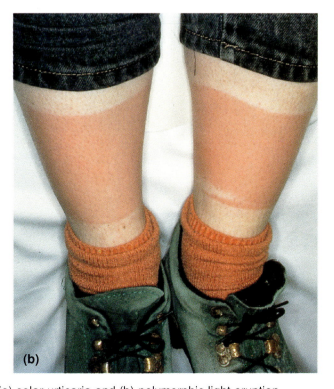

Fig. 4.18 Inducing clinically diagnostic lesions in (a) solar urticaria and (b) polymorphic light eruption.

PHOTOPROVOCATION TESTS

Patients with PLE frequently present in the absence of a diagnostic rash. In this situation it is convenient to induce lesions, confirming that the patient is photosensitive and in some situations inducing clinically diagnostic lesions (Fig. 4.18). The principle followed is that of repeatedly exposing the patient to a given dose of broad-band UV, usually 70% of the pretested MED, with either UVB or UVA or with a solar simulator which delivers at high intensity a spectral mix equivalent to that received from sun exposure at midday in summer. UVA is more successful in inducing PLE compared with UVB; 60% of patients with PLE are UVA-sensitive, an additional 25% appear to be both UVB- and UVA-sensitive and very few react to UVB alone. Solar urticaria is readily provoked by broad-band UV irradiation, and in some patients only broad-band radiation induces lesions and MITs may be normal. In hydroa vacciniforme (Fig. 4.19) – a very rare photosensitive disease leading to blistering and scarring of the skin – diagnostic lesions may be induced both clinically and histologically.

Drug-induced phototoxicity and photoallergy

Phototoxic reactions depend on a direct interaction of UV radiation or visible light with the drug or chemical in the skin, with or without oxygen,

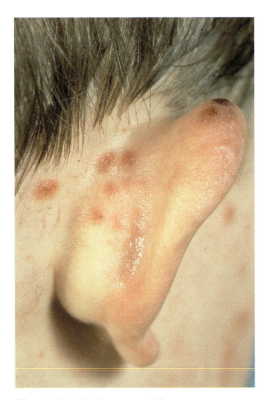

Fig. 4.19 Hydroa vacciniforme.

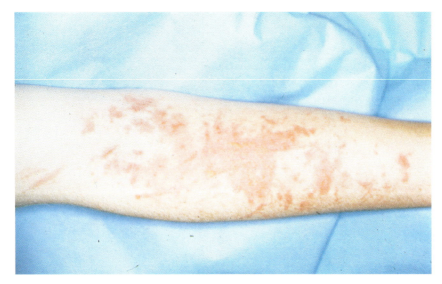

Fig. 4.20 Phytophotodermatitis.

without an allergic reaction. Inflammatory effects are mediated in a variety of ways, including intercalation and alteration of DNA in the case of psoralens encountered therapeutically as photosensitizing drugs for PUVA therapy, or inadvertently as a consequence of contact with psoralens in plants (phytophotodermatitis; Fig. 4.20). Drug-induced photoallergy is much less common and difficult to document. Chlorpromazine, sulphonamides and possibly thiazides may lead to both photoallergic and phototoxic reactions.

FURTHER READING

Cerio R and Jackson WF. *A Colour Atlas of Allergic Skin Disorders*. Wolfe, London, 1992.

Cronin E. *Contact Dermatitis.* Churchill Livingstone, Edinburgh, 1980.

Dahl MV and Lynch PJ (eds) *Current Opinion in Dermatology 1994*. Current Science, Philadelphia, 1994, pp. 175–193.

Hawk JLM (ed) *Seminars in Dermatology*. 1990; **9**: 1–77.

Roitt I. Brostoff J and Male D (eds) *Immunology.* Churchill Livingstone, Edinburgh, 1985.

Chapter 5

Bacteriology and mycology

John P. Leeming, Elizabeth M. Johnson and David W. Warnock

The diagnosis of bacterial and fungal infections depends upon a combination of clinical observation and laboratory investigation. Superficial bacterial and fungal infections often produce characteristic lesions which suggest the diagnosis, but laboratory input can aid the diagnostic process where this is not the case, either because several microorganisms and/or non-infective processes produce similar clinical pictures, or because the appearance of a lesion has been rendered atypical by previous treatment. Furthermore, microbiology laboratories can identify the presence of antibiotic-resistant organisms and can be useful in monitoring the response to treatment, particularly where clinical resolution tends to lag behind microbial eradication (e.g. nail infections).

The successful laboratory diagnosis of bacterial or fungal infection depends in large part on the collection of appropriate clinical specimens for investigation. It is also dependent on the selection of appropriate microbiological test procedures. These differ from one infection to another, and depend on the site of infection as well as the presenting symptoms and clinical signs (Tables 5.1–5.3).

COLLECTION OF SPECIMENS

To establish or confirm the diagnosis of suspected bacterial or fungal infection, it is essential for the clinician to provide the laboratory with adequate specimens for investigation. Inappropriate collection, storage or processing of specimens can result in a missed diagnosis. Moreover, to ensure that the most appropriate laboratory tests are performed, it is essential for the clinician to indicate that a bacterial or fungal infection is suspected and to provide sufficient background information. In addition to specifying the source of the specimen, it is important to provide information on any underlying illness, recent antimicrobial therapy, recent travel or previous residence abroad, any animal contacts and the patient's occupation. This information will help the laboratory to anticipate which pathogens are most likely to be involved and permit the selection of the most relevant test procedures.

A Wood's lamp (a portable source of long-wave ultraviolet light) can be useful for the selection of sites of active infection, especially where lesions are inconspicuous or atypical. When shone on hair infected with certain dermatophyte species, an apple-green fluorescence is observed, while pityriasisversicolor lesions often produce greenish, golden-yellow or pinkish fluorescence and erythrasma a coral-red fluorescence. This phenomenon, discussed further in Chapter 1, can also be used in the laboratory to aid the differentiation of dermatophytes.

Contamination of samples by saprophytic skin flora may mask the presence of pathogens, particularly slow-growing fungi, in subsequent cultures. Cleansing the skin with 70% alcohol will both remove and kill many superficial bacteria and this procedure is often helpful when examining cutaneous and scalp lesions (and sometimes nails) for fungal infection. Use of alcohol is not indicated when sampling superficial lesions of probable bacterial aetiology, but is helpful before other samples are taken. Prior cleaning is also useful for the removal of ointments, creams or powders applied to lesions which may interfere with microscopy and culture.

Apart from specimens from cases of suspected dermatophytosis (which can be stored for days or even weeks before processing), specimens for microbiological investigation must be processed as soon as possible after collection. Delay may result in the death of fastidious organisms, in overgrowth of contaminants, and/or multiplication in the number of organisms present.

Swabs

Although swabs are frequently employed as a convenient method for the collection of material, they are only suitable for superficial bacterial infections such as impetigo; swabs of the skin surface overlying an infection of the dermis are unlikely to be productive. Where swabs are employed, moistening the tip with sterile water or saline will increase the yield of organisms and the

Table 5.1 Aetiology of some bacterial infections on the skin

Disease	Causative organism	Comments
Erythrasma	*Corynebacterium minutissimum*	Coral-pink fluorescence under Wood's light
Trichomycosis axillaris/pubis	Various coryneform bacteria	Atypical growth of normal skin bacteria
Impetigo	Group A β-haemolytic streptococci, *Staphylococcus aureus*	
Folliculitis	*Staphylococcus aureus*	Rarely Gram-negative bacillus superinfection of antibiotic-treated acne or immersion in contaminated water (especially *Pseudomonas aeruginosa*)
Furuncules, styes	*Staphylococcus aureus*	
Paronychia (acute)	*Staphylococcus aureus* group A β-haemolytic streptococci	*Candida albicans* more common in chronic paronychias
Fish-tank granuloma	*Mycobacterium marinum*	
Ecthyma	*Staphylococcus aureus* group A β-haemolytic streptococci	
Ecthyma gangrenosum	*Pseudomonas aeruginosa,* other Gram-negative bacilli	Affects immunocompromised patients who may suffer similar invasive infection with various fungi
Erysipelas	Group A β-haemolytic streptococci	
Erysipeloid	*Erysipelothrix rhusiopathiae*	Veterinary pathogen acquired by occupational contact with fish or meat
Cellulitis*	Group A β-haemolytic strepto-cocci, *Staphylococcus aureus*	*Haemophilus influenzae* can cause facial cellulitis in young children
Necrotizing fasciitis* (streptococcal gangrene)	Group A β-haemolytic streptococci, often with *Staphylococcus aureus*	
Synergistic necrotizing fasciitis*	Mixed cultures, frequently anaerobic and microaerophilic cocci, *Bacteroides* or *Fusobacterium* spp.	
Progressive bacterial synergistic (Meleney's) gangrene*	Anaerobic or microaerophilic coccus plus aerobe (often *Staphylococcus aureus*)	Clinically similar disease caused by *Entamoeba histolytica*
Clostridial cellulitis gas gangrene*	*Clostridium* spp., usually mixed cultures	
Membranous ulcer	*Corynebacterium diphtheriae* usually mixed	Usually acquired during foreign travel
Erythema chronicum migrans (Lyme disease)	*Borrelia burgdorferi*	Microscopy and culture are insensitive; serology is useful but antibody response can be slow (≥ 6 weeks)
Secondary infections Infected eczema	*Staphylococcus aureus*	
Ulcers and burns	Many species, including *Staphylococcus aureus.* Group A β-haemolytic streptococci and anaerobes	Interpret culture results with caution: many organisms are saprophytic rather than pathogenic in this setting

*Note that organisms are difficult to isolate from many infections of the dermis. Diagnosis is therefore normally made on clinical grounds. Although the subdivisions used here are widely employed, a spectrum of disease is observed both clinically and microbiologically.

Table 5.2 Non-dermatophyte causes of superficial mycoses

Disease	Causative organism	Clinical features
Pityriasis versicolor	*Malassezia furfur*	Brown-coloured scaly macules on trunk, back and upper arms; hypopigmented lesions on dark skin
Tinea nigra	*Exophiala werneckii*	Smooth, brown, irregularly pigmented patches on palms, sometimes feet
Black piedra	*Piedraon hortae*	Dark brown/black gritty nodules on scalp hair
White piedra	*Trichosporum beigelii*	Pale, soft nodules on beard, axillary or pubic hairs
Onychomycosis	*Scopulariopsis brevicaulis*, *Acremonium* spp., *Fusarium* spp., *Aspergillus* spp	Brown discoloration, crumbling nail plate, white patches; toe nails more frequently affected
Scytalidium infection	*Scytalidium dimidiatum* (*Hendersonula toruloidea*), *Scytalidium hyalinum*	Chronic infection of soles, palms and nails resembling dermatophyte infection; brown discoloration of nails, subungual hyperkeratosis
Candidosis	*Candida albicans*, other *Candida* spp.	Erythematous infection of intertriginous areas of skin; paronychia; onychia; infection of mucous membranes
Mycetoma	*Exophiala* spp., *Leptosphaeria senegalis Madurella* spp., *Pyrenochaeta* spp., *Scedosporium* spp.	Draining sinus tracts, grains (white or yellow to black), tumefaction

swab must be transported to the laboratory in transport medium, which is provided with the swab by many manufacturers.

Skin scrapings and strippings

For the majority of fungal infections tissue specimens are preferred. Skin, nail and hair specimens for mycological examination should be collected into folded squares of black paper (about 10 cm × 10 cm). The use of paper permits the specimen to dry out, which helps reduce bacterial contamination and also provides a convenient means of storing specimens for long periods (12 months or longer). Material should be collected from cutaneous lesions by scraping outwards from the margin of the lesion with the edge of a glass microscope slide or a blunt scalpel. Samples collected from the edge of a spreading lesion are more likely to yield viable organisms than material from the centre of the lesion. If there is minimal scaling, as often occurs with lesions of the glabrous skin, it is helpful to use clear adhesive tape to remove material for examination. The adhesive strip should be pressed against the lesion, peeled off and placed, adhesive side down, on a clean glass microscope slide for transportation to the laboratory.

Nail specimens

Nail specimens should be taken from any discoloured, dystrophic or brittle parts of the nail. Specimens should be cut as far back as possible from the edge of the nail and should include the full thickness of the nail because some fungi are confined to the lower parts. If distal subungual lesions are present, use a currette, spatula or nail elevator to obtain debris from under the distal edge of the nail. If there is superficial nail plate involvement, take thin superficial scrapings with a curette, scalpel or nail elevator. If there is proximal subungual involvement, a nail drill or scalpel may be used to obtain debris. Pus may be obtained from under the nailfold by applying light pressure.

Hair samples

Specimens from the scalp should include hair roots, the contents of plugged follicles and skin scales. Hairs should be plucked from the scalp with forceps. Cut hairs without roots are unsuitable for mycological investigation because the infection is usually confined near or below the surface of the scalp. As mentioned previously, a Wood's light can be of value in selecting infected hairs. Another technique which is useful for collection of material from patients with incon-

spicuous scalp lesions is hairbrush sampling. The scalp is brushed with a plastic hairbrush or scalp massage pad which is then pressed into the surface of an agar plate. The brushes or pads can be sterilized in 1% chlorhexidine for 1 h, rinsed in sterile water and dried before being reused.

Pus, aspirates and biopsies

To detect more deep-seated bacterial and fungal infections, aspirates of pus or bullous fluid or biopsy specimens may be necessary. Pus from undrained abscesses or sinus tracts should be collected with a sterile needle and syringe. If any grains are visible in the pus (as in mycetoma), these must be collected. Needle aspirates of saline (0.1–0.2 ml) injected into vasculitic skin lesions

Table 5.3 Mode of infection of some common dermatophytes

Organism	Natural reservoir	Usual sites	Hair invasion
Trichophyton erinacei	Hedgehogs	Scalp, hands, limbs	
T. mentagrophytes	Rodents	Hands, limbs, nails	Large-spored ectothrix (3–5 μm)
T. mentagrophytes var. interdigitale	Humans	Feet, nails	
T. rubrum	Humans	Hands, feet, nails, trunk, groin, limbs, face, scalp	
T. schoenleinii	Humans	Scalp	Endothrix*
T. soudanense	Humans	Scalp, limbs	Endothrix
T. tonsurans	Humans	Scalp, face	Endothrix
T. verrucosum	Cattle	Scalp, neck, face, limbs	Large-spored ectothrix (5–10 μm)
T. violaceum	Humans	Scalp, limbs	Endothrix
Microsporum audouinii	Humans	Scalp, limbs	Small-spored ectothrix (2–3 μm)*
M. canis	Dogs, cats	Scalp, face, neck, hands, limbs,	Small-spored ecothrix (2–3 μm)*
M. equinum	Horses	Face, hands, limbs	Small-spored ectothrix (2–3 μm)*
M. gypseum	Soil	Hands, limbs	Small-spored ectothrix (2–3 μm)*
Epidermophyton floccosum	Humans	Groin, hands, feet	

* Fluorescent under Wood's light

associated with suspected meningococcal infection can be productive, but similar samples taken from areas of cellulitis produce a low yield of pathogens. Biopsies of deep active lesional tissue can be used by microbiologists for culture and by histopathologists for microscopic visualization of organisms in stained tissue sections. Separate specimens are required for each purpose; histopathology specimens transported in formol-saline are unsuitable for microbiology.

Blood

Blood cultures are indicated when infection is deep-seated and the patient is systemically unwell. The venepuncture site should be rubbed vigorously with an alcohol-based disinfectant for 20–30s and allowed to dry before drawing blood. Pairs of bottles containing the liquid medium into which the blood is to be injected are provided by the receiving laboratory. The bottles, one for aerobic and one for anaerobic incubation, are now likely to be commercially prepared for use in one of several automated laboratory systems. The volume of blood accepted by these bottles varies, but will be stated on the labels. Organisms are usually present in blood at low concentration and therefore the recovery rate will be improved if more than one pair of bottles is inoculated, preferably by separate venepuncture. Most authorities recommend a maximum of three pairs.

Blood should also be collected for serological examinations if Lyme disease or treponemal infection (yaws or syphilis) is suspected, and for antistreptolysin O and antistreptodornase titres in cases of cellulitis and fasciitis (see later).

LABORATORY DIAGNOSIS OF BACTERIAL AND FUNGAL INFECTIONS

Direct microscopic examination

The direct microscopic examination of clinical material is one of the simpler and most helpful procedures for the laboratory diagnosis of infection. Various methods can be used; unstained wet-mount preparations may be examined by light-field, dark-field or phase-contrast illumination; or dried smears can be stained and examined.

BACTERIAL INFECTION

The Gram stain is the commonest preparation used for bacteriological microscopy. Various modifications can be used for visualization of bacteria in tissues and their subdivision into Gram-positive (retain primary stain; usually violet) or Gram-negative (do not retain primary stain and therefore are the colour of the secondary stain, usually pink or green), and into morphological groups. This rarely provides a definite diagnosis because Gram morphology is not sufficiently differential to discriminate between different pathogens or between pathogens and non-pathogens in contaminated specimens.

FUNGAL INFECTION

To facilitate microscopic examination of skin, hair and nail samples for fungal hyphae, they are softened by the application of 20–30% potassium hydroxide (KOH). A few drops of KOH are placed on tissue fragments on a glass microscope slide and covered with a coverslip. After 10–20 min the coverslip can be squashed down by applying gentle pressure to yield a single layer of cells in which fungal hyphae can be more easily differentiated. These are septate, regular in width and often show branching; there may also be chains of arthrospores (Fig. 5.1). Particular care should be taken with samples of hair so that the arrangement of spores is not disturbed.

Although specific staining is not usually necessary, stains such as Chlorazol black E, Parker's Quink blue-black ink or Calcofluor white may help to differentiate hyphae from common artefacts such as clothes fibres and 'mosaic fungus' in which deposition of cholesterol and other substances around the periphery of cells resembles chains of arthrospores.

The microscopic recognition of fungal hyphae and/or arthrospores in clinical material is sufficient for the diagnosis of dermatophytosis. With hair, the size and disposition of the arthrospores also give some indication as to the species of fungus involved. Arthrospores are usually described as small or large (2–4 μm or up to 10 μm in diameter respectively) and to be either ectothrix or endothrix (outside or inside the infected hair; Table 5.3).

Parker's ink (in equal volume with 30% KOH) and 1% crystal violet in water are particularly useful stains for demonstrating *Malassezia furfur* (*Pityrosporum* spp.) in scales from pityriasis versicolor. On direct microscopic examination *M. furfur* appears as clusters of yeast cells together with short broad filaments which are seldom branched (Fig. 5.2). Because this appearance is pathognomonic of pityriasis versicolor, and because *M. furfur* also lives saprophytically on the skin of most adults, confirmation by culture is not helpful. In other conditions associated with *M. furfur*, including seborrhoeic dermatitis and malassezia folliculitis, this characteristic morphology is not observed and the diagnosis must be made clinically, although microscopic observation of numerous yeasts in either expressed follicular contents or biopsy sections may be helpful.

Culture

Culture permits the species of pathogen involved to be determined, and can therefore provide information as to the source of the infection and aid the selection of the most appropriate form of treatment. Culture also provides the material necessary for further laboratory investigations, such as antibiotic susceptibility testing.

The great majority of cultures are made on the surface of nutrient media solidified with agar (agar plates). The composition of these media depends on the organisms to be cultured and often includes components to stimulate the growth of expected pathogens and to inhibit the growth of other microorganisms. Selection of the appropriate incubation temperature, period and atmosphere is also important for the successful isolation of individual pathogens. It is therefore essential that the clinician provides adequate clinical information on request forms and informs the laboratory if a particular infection is suspected, permitting selection of the most appropriate culture procedures, which will often include several different culture media and incubation regimens.

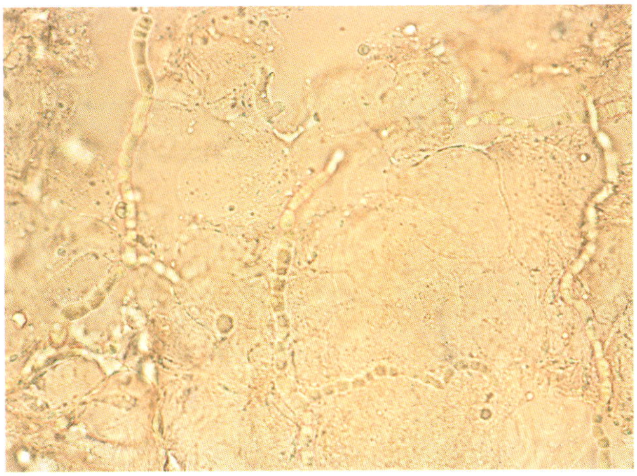

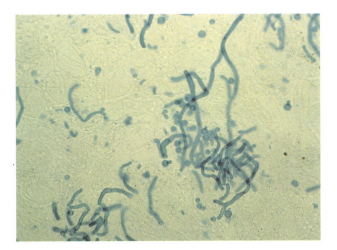

Fig. 5.1 Unstained potassium hydroxide preparation of skin demonstrating presence of dermatophyte hyphae, some of which are fragmenting into arthrospores.

Fig. 5.2 *Malassezia furfur* in a skin preparation stained with equal volumes of blue-black Parker Quink ink and 20% potassium hydroxide. Note the appearance of short, slightly curved, unbranched hyphae and the presence of yeast forms.

BACTERIAL ISOLATION

The most important bacteriological culture medium is the blood agar plate. Enrichment with blood encourages the growth of many of the more demanding bacteria and the extent of haemolysis around colonies is an important guide to the identity of some groups, most notably the streptococci (Figs 5.3–5.5). Incubation of these plates in carbon dioxide-enriched and oxygen-free environments permits the recovery of capnocytophagic (carbon dioxide-dependent) and anaerobic bacteria; incorporation of narrow-spectrum antibiotics suppresses growth of contaminants. MacConkey's bile salts–lactose agar is useful for the isolation and identification of less demanding organisms, particularly *Pseudomonas aeruginosa*, coliforms and other enteric bacteria.

FUNGAL ISOLATION

Most pathogenic fungi are not particularly nutritionally demanding, but the development of spores and other structures used for their differentiation is medium-dependent. Mycologists vary in their preferences but Sabouraud's glucose–peptone agar is widely employed for primary isolation of yeasts and filamentous fungi. Bacterial growth is suppressed by incorporating a broad-spectrum antibiotic such as chloramphenicol (50 mg/l, 0.005%). Dermatophytes are often cultured on media containing cycloheximide (Actidione; 500 mg/l, 0.05%), but media without this selective agent must also be used if other fungi are included in the differential diagnosis. It is not unusual to isolate moulds other than dermatophytes from abnormal skin and

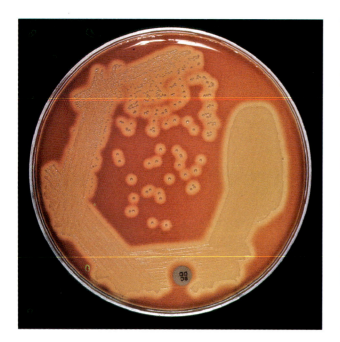

Fig. 5.3 A culture of a Lancefield group A β-haemolytic streptococcus (*Streptococcus pyogenes*) on blood agar. Note the zone of complete clearing around colonies produced by the action of bacterial haemolysins. The antibiotic disc contains bacitracin which is sometimes used to differentiate *Streptococcus pyogenes* (sensitive) from other β-haemolytic streptococci (resistant).

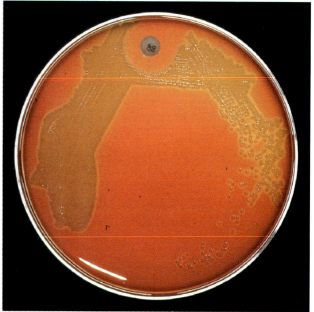

Fig. 5.4 A culture of *Streptococcus pneumoniae*, an α-haemolytic streptococcus, on blood agar. Contrast the zone of incomplete clearing and green discoloration typical of α-haemolytic streptococci with β-haemolysis shown in Figure 5.3. The antibiotic disc contains optochin which is commonly used to differentiate *Streptococcus pneumoniae* (sensitive) from other α-haemolytic (viridans) streptococci (resistant).

nails. In many cases, these are casual, transient contaminants and direct microscopic examination of clinical material is negative. However, certain moulds (e.g. *Scopulariopsis brevicaulis* and *Scytalidium dimidiatum*) are capable of causing infection and when this is so, it is important that their significance is recognized.

The isolation and identification of a mycelial fungus can take several weeks because of their slow rates of growth. In such unavoidable instances, the result may become available too late either to help with the diagnosis or with the choice of treatment. Nevertheless, culture should always be attempted so that a definite diagnosis can be obtained.

Identification

Experienced microbiologists can identify many bacterial isolates to genus and sometimes species level simply by their appearance on isolation plates (Figs 5.3–5.5). This process is often aided by the microscopic examination of a Gram-stained smear of cultured material (Figs 5.6 and 5.7). For

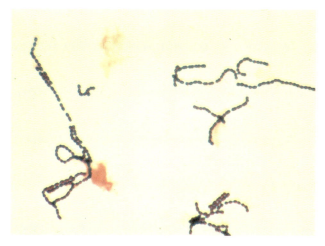

Fig. 5.6 Typical appearance of streptococci in Gram-stained film. These were taken directly from a blood culture bottle. Note the production of chain of cells (1–2 µm in diameter) which are often slightly elongated along the axis of the chain. *Streptococcus pneumoniae* differs in that cells usually appear in pairs (diplococci).

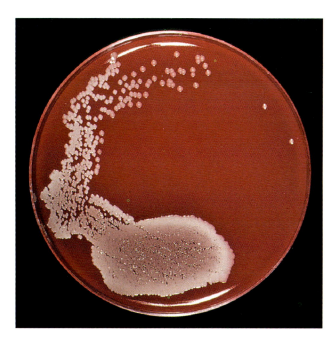

Fig. 5.5 A culture of *Staphylococcus aureus* on blood agar. Note that after overnight incubation the colonies are larger and more opaque than streptococci but marked pigmentation is unusual. The golden-yellow pigmentation responsible for the species name is observed if plates are reincubated, particularly at room temperature.

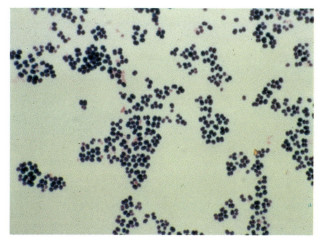

Fig. 5.7 Typical appearance of staphylococci in Gram-stained film. Cells are usually a little larger than streptococci and are arranged in two-dimensional clusters.

hyphal fungi, examination of the macroscopic morphology of the culture, particularly the production of pigment, is helpful (Fig. 5.8) but it is also important to examine the microscopic morphology, in particularly the spore-bearing structures. The three genera of dermatophytes, *Trichophyton, Microsporum* and *Epidermophyton*, and many pathogenic species of the first two genera have a distinctive microscopic morphology (Figs 5.9 and 5.10). However further investigations are frequently required to assign isolates to clinically relevant taxa. For many yeasts and bacteria identification requires biochemical characterization, e.g. the utilization and/or production of acid from sugars and various other organic substrates. Several manufacturers have incorporated the most useful biochemical tests into multicompartment test modules, with interpretation facilitated by a change in colour of chromogenic substrates or pH indicators (Fig. 5.11). The availability of these kits has greatly expanded the range of microorganisms readily identified by hospital laboratories.

Some specific tests used for organisms of dermatological importance are worthy of particular note because they are often used to define a pathogenic group. Staphylococci are divided by their ability to clot plasma into the pathogenic coagulase-positive isolates (*Staphylococcus aureus*) and coagulase-negative staphylococci of low pathogenicity (formerly known as *S. albus* but now subdivided into many species, including *S. epidermidis, S. capitis, S. hominis* and *S. haemolyticis*). The β-haemolytic streptococci (those which produce a zone of complete clearing around colonies on blood agar) are divided according to the presence of antigens in their cell walls into Lancefield groups. Group A (*Streptococcus pyogenes*) accounts for the great majority of streptococcal infections of the skin. Kits for the rapid extraction and agglutination of the relevant antigens permit the rapid identification of the most common human pathogenic groups (A–D, F, G; Fig. 5.12).

Yeasts are commonly divided into those which are germ tube-positive (most *Candida albicans* isolates) and those which are germ tube-negative.

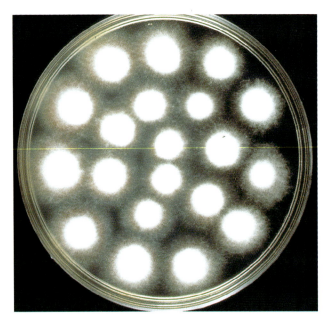

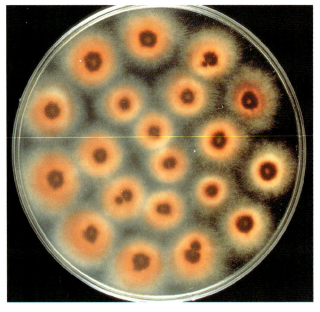

Fig. 5.8 Typical morphology of *Trichophyton rubrum* on glucose–peptone agar plate. (a) Top view; (b) reverse of the plate shows the production of the characteristic red-brown pigment from which the organism gets its name.

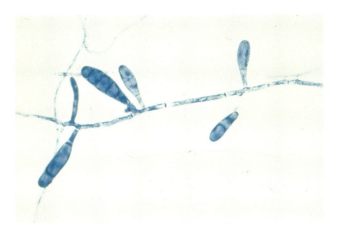

Fig. 5.9 Lactophenol cotton-blue stain of *Epidermophyton floccosum* showing characteristic club-shaped macroconidia approximately 30 µm in length. Microconidia are not produced by this species.

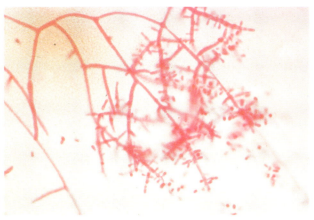

Fig. 5.10 Lactofuchsin stain of *Trichophyton erinacei* showing characteristic club-shaped microconidia borne along the sides and ends of branched hyphae.

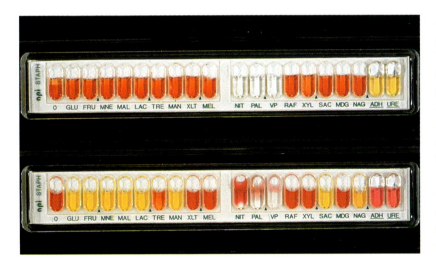

Fig. 5.11 Identification of microorganisms by biochemical characterization. This is a *Staphylococcus aureus* isolate in a commercially produced gallery of biochemical tests (API Staph, bioMérieux). The upper strip has just been inoculated with a suspension of the test strain; the bottom strip has been incubated for 18 h and reagents added to wells 11–13. Similar kits are available from several manufacturers for the speciation of many genera of bacteria and yeasts.

Fig. 5.12 Lancefield antigenic grouping of β-haemolytic streptococci. Antigens are now usually extracted from the cell walls of isolates using enzymatic preparations. Drops of group-specific antisera, in this case bound to latex particles, are then mixed with the extract. Visualization of agglutination is aided by the latex. Drop 1 contains group A-specific antiserum (positive); the other drops contain group B-, C-, D-, F- and G-specific antiserum respectively (all negative). This test was performed using a Streptex kit (Murex Diagnostics).

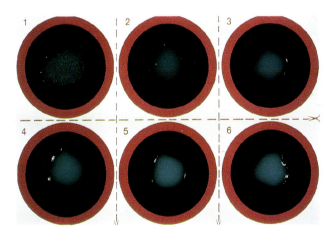

75

This is determined by incubating a dilute suspension of yeast in serum for 2–4 h and examining for outgrowths of germ tubes (short hyphae) microscopically (Fig. 5.13). Although germ tube-negative yeasts are less pathogenic, they should nevertheless be identified to species level if suspected of contributing to a disease process because they may vary in their susceptibility to antifungal drugs (see below).

OTHER LABORATORY INVESTIGATIONS

Antibiotic susceptibilities

The susceptibility of a microorganism can sometimes be deduced without further investigation once its identity is known. Thus, most fungal infections of the skin are treated empirically and treatment modification is likely to be necessary only in the case of treatment failure or the isolation of a less common organism known to be intrinsically resistant to the treatment selected. With bacteria the prediction of susceptibility is less straightforward because of the widespread distribution of acquired resistance genes.

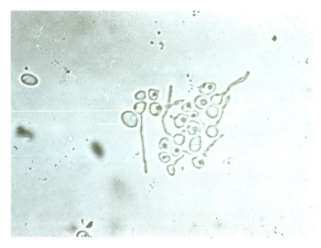

Fig. 5.13 Germ tubes of *Candida albicans* formed after 3 h incubation in horse serum at 37°C. These should not be confused with the pseudomycelium formed by other *Candida* spp., where there is pinching in at the point of origin and at septa along the hyphae.

Although group A β-haemolytic streptococci can be assumed to be susceptible to penicillins, their sensitivity to tetracyclines and macrolides can no longer be taken for granted and laboratory confirmation is important. Rates of resistance of staphylococci to these agents are much higher, with the spread of methicillin-resistant *Staphylococcus aureus* (MRSA) posing a particular problem.

The most common method of determining the susceptibility of bacteria is to place antibiotic-impregnated discs on agar plates evenly inoculated with a suspension of the test bacterium. After incubation the resultant 'lawn' of bacterial growth is interrupted by zones of inhibition around the antibiotics to which the organism is sensitive. Sensitive control strains may or may not be included on the same plate (Stokes and Kirby-Bauer procedures respectively); whichever technique is used, this approach is versatile, cheap and easy to set up and interpret if properly standardized (Fig. 5.14). Another approach is to define a concentration of an antibiotic to which an organism should be susceptible if therapy is likely to be successful. When antibiotic is incorporated into agar plates at this 'breakpoint' concentration, sensitive isolates fail to grow on the surface while resistant isolates produce visible colonies. This technique is more successful than disc-testing for hydrophobic agents, including many antifungals, which fail to diffuse well in agar.

Determination of the **minimum inhibitory concentration** (MIC) and/or **minimum lethal/cidal concentration** of an agent for an organism gives a more precise measure of that organism's susceptibility. This is achieved by making twofold dilutions of the antibiotic in either culture broth or molten agar medium immediately before pouring plates. After inoculation and incubation of the resultant series of broths or plates, the MIC is defined as the lowest concentration of the antibiotic which completely inhibits the (visible) growth of the organism. If broths are used, the minimum cidal concentration of the drug can be determined by subculturing a small volume of each broth on to antibiotic-free medium; organisms which have been inhibited, but not killed,

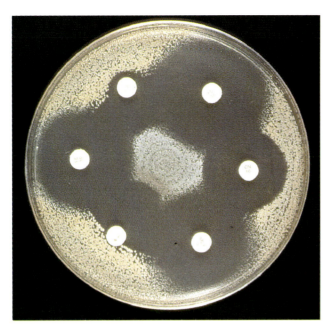

Fig. 5.14 Disc diffusion antibiotic susceptibility performed by a modification of the Stokes comparative technique. A turntable rotates the plate to aid inoculation of the central area with a swab moistened in a dilute suspension of a sensitive control strain. The outer annular area is similarly inoculated with the isolate to be tested and antibiotic discs are placed between. Zones of inhibition are usually read after overnight incubation. This *Staphylococcus aureus* isolate is resistant to penicillin G (P) and erythromycin (E) but sensitive to tetracycline (T), fusidic acid (FD), gentamicin (CN) and mupirocin (MUP).

treatment. Tests are often conducted using a modification of the broth-based MIC method described above. Experience has shown that with these agents the concentration producing complete inhibition of growth is not usually a clinically useful cut-off point. The lowest concentration at which growth (measured in a photometer) fails to reach a pre-selected percentage (often 30 or 50%) of an antibiotic-free control is the preferred end-point (Fig. 5.15).

Epidemiological typing of isolates

Occasionally it is desirable for epidemiological purposes to determine whether two or more isolates of similar organisms are likely to have originated from a common source. Examples of such an occasion would be a cluster of infections which appeared to be associated with a health care institution, or the investigation of an atopic

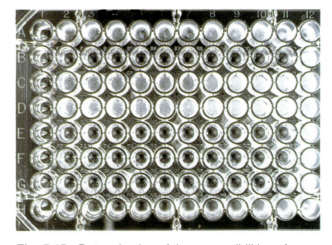

Fig. 5.15 Determination of the susceptibilities of yeasts to antifungal drugs performed in microtitre plates (the broth microdilution method). Wells contain doubling dilutions of antifungal drugs from left to right. The lowest drug concentration at which there is 50% or more inhibition of growth as compared to the drug-free control (column 12) is determined by photometry. The test if often performed on a larger scale in test tubes (the broth macrodilution method). Note that when determining bacterial minimum inhibitory concentrations, complete inhibition of growth is taken as the end-point (see text).

will produce visible growth. These methods are time-consuming and are usually reserved for serious or problematic infections. Modifications of these procedures can be used to assess interactions between antibiotics when the use of multiple antibiotics is desirable.

In some yeast species, notably *Candida albicans*, acquisition of resistance to azole antifungals has been observed during prolonged treatment (note that some other *Candida* species, including *C. glabrata* and *C. krusei*, are intrinsically less susceptible to some azoles, particularly fluconazole). Antifungal susceptibility testing may therefore contribute to the selection of appropriate therapy when infection is protracted or refractory to azole dermatitis patient who suffers repeated re-infection with *S. aureus* despite apparently successful antibiotic treatment. For this purpose the subdivision of a species into subgroups or strains is necessary.

For *S. aureus* this is usually done by determining the phage (bacteriophage) group of isolates. Bacteriophages are viruses of bacteria and they are frequently able to infect only subgroups of a species which carry a specific surface receptor molecule to which they have evolved to attach. The phage group of an isolate of *S. aureus* is defined by its susceptibility to lysis by a standard panel of phages with different specificities. Group A β-haemolytic streptococci are commonly typed by extraction and serological characterization of families of antigenically heterogeneous proteins (M and T antigens) from their cell walls.

The development of methods for the genetic 'fingerprinting' of organisms is revolutionizing our approach to typing bacteria and fungi, an increasing proportion of which can be characterized in this manner by reference laboratories.

The typing of dermatophyte isolates has seldom been attempted, but useful epidemiological information can be gathered by identifying the infecting species. Dermatophytes are termed geophilic, zoophilic or anthropophilic depending on whether their normal habitat is the soil, an animal or humans (Table 5.3). These different natural reservoirs have important epidemiological implications in relation to the acquisition, site and spread of human infection.

Other diagnostic approaches

SEROLOGY

Serological diagnosis is rarely indicated in superficial infections of the skin, but can be valuable in deeper infection, especially those in which the probability of making a diagnosis by culture is low (e.g. cellulitis, Lyme disease, syphilis, mycetoma and sporotrichosis). It is necessary to collect both acute and convalescent sera in order to observe conversion of immunoglobulin M (IgM) to IgG and/or rising antibody titres which characterize many infections and to help differentiate current from past infection.

HISTOPATHOLOGY

Histological examination of biopsied material is frequently helpful in the diagnosis of invasive infection, e.g. Grocott silver stain for visualizing invasive fungi in tissue sections. Immunofluorescent staining of frozen sections has been advocated as a sensitive method for the detection of streptococci in the dermis but this service is not widely available. Biopsies for immunofluorescent staining should be snap-frozen rather than formolized.

NEW TECHNOLOGY

New diagnostic tests are constantly being developed. Notable among the methods currently being developed is the detection of microorganisms by polymerase chain reaction or gene probes. These are very sensitive methods of detecting specific lengths of DNA unique to the pathogen under investigation (Chapter 9). These procedures are largely experimental and therefore not widely available currently. However, they are likely to be introduced increasingly into the repertoire of larger laboratories for diagnoses which are at present problematic.

FURTHER READING

Murray PR, Baron EJ, Pfaller MA, Tenover FC and Yolken RH (eds) *Manual of Clinical Microbiology,* 6th edn. American Society for Microbiology, Washington DC, 1995.

Evans EGV and Richardson MD (eds) *Medical Mycology: A Practical Approach.* IRL Press at Oxford University Press, Oxford, 1989.

Hawkey PM and Lewis DA (eds) *Medical Bacteriology: a Practical Approach.* IRL Press at Oxford University Press, Oxford, 1989

Kwon-Chung KJ and Bennett JE. *Medical Mycology.* 4th edn. Lea & Febiger, Philadelphia, 1992.

Mandell GL, Bennett JE and Dohn R (eds) *Principles and Practice of Infectious Diseases*, 4th edn. Churchill Livingstone, New York, 1995.

Richardson MD and Warnock DW. *Fungal Infection: Diagnosis and Management.* 2nd edn. Blackwell Scientific Publications, Oxford, 1997.

Chapter 6

Tests for viral, HIV-related and tropical skin infections

Dee Anna Glaser and Neal S. Penneys

■ **Viral infections**
Human papillomavirus (HPV)
Poxviruses
Viral exanthems
Herpesviruses
HIV
   Primary HIV infection

■ **HIV-related infections**
Syphilis
Chancroid
Gonorrhoea
Herpes infections
   Herpes simplex virus (HSV)
   Varicella-zoster virus (VZV)
   Cytomegalovirus (CMV)
   Epstein–Barr virus
Bacillary angiomatosis
Mycobacteria

■ **Tropical infections**
Leprosy
Leishmaniasis
Coccidioidomycosis
Cryptococcosis
Histoplasmosis
Onchocerciasis
Trichinosis

This chapter will discuss the clinical investigation, when necessary, of viral infections in immunocompetent individuals before focusing on HIV and HIV-related infections. Space does not allow a comprehensive account of tropical diseases but investigation of some of the more important tropical skin infections is reviewed here.

VIRAL INFECTIONS

Most of the common viral skin infections are recognizable by clinical presentation and extensive investigations will not be necessary. This is true for viral warts (caused by human papillomavirus), molluscum contagiosum warts, human orf, viral exanthems such as measles, roseola, rubella and erythema infectiosum (fifth disease), and herpes simplex or varicella infections. Investigations are required when the clinical features are less obvious, as one sees, for example, in infectious mononucleosis, caused by the Epstein–Barr virus.

Human papillomavirus (HPV)

Various DNA subtypes of HPV can be identified by the polymerase chain reaction (PCR) but this test is usually not necessary with common viral warts. Genital infection with HPV 16 and 18 carries a risk of malignant change and some squamous carcinomas in renal transplant recipients contain oncogenic HPV. Similarly, individuals with epidermodysplasia verruciformis have numerous premalignant HPV-induced warts. In difficult cases, histological examination of skin biopsies will usually confirm the presence of HPV. In addition, antibodies for immunohistochemical labelling are commercially available.

Poxviruses

The clinical appearance of molluscum contagiosum warts is generally characteristic but in doubtful cases Tzanck smears and/or histological examination (see Chapter 2) may be diagnostic. Patients with HIV are more prone to infection with molluscum contagiosum warts which, in this setting, may persist despite treatment.

Human orf is a contagious vesicular disease caused by a parapoxvirus, contracted from direct contact with infected sheep or goats. The diagnosis may be confirmed histologically or by demonstration of the poxvirus by electron microscopy.

Viral exanthems

In infections for which serology is available, two specimens of clotted blood should be taken to be certain of a diagnosis. The first sample is taken soon after the onset of symptoms, before significant antibody production has occurred. The second sample is usually taken 10 days later, but may be sooner (e.g. 5 days) in rubella. A fourfold or greater rise in titre between acute and convalescent sera is generally accepted as diagnostic.

The demonstration of specific immunoglobulin M (IgM) or IgA antibody in a single acute serum can be of diagnostic value in rubella. However, serological responses to viral infections are often unpredictable in HIV-infected individuals.

Herpes viruses

The clinical diagnosis of herpes simplex virus and varicella virus infections is not usually difficult. The investigation of these and other herpesvirus infections in the context of HIV infection is discussed in some detail below.

Infectious mononucleosis (glandular fever) is diagnosed by examination of a blood film for abnormal lymphocytes. The Paul–Bunnell test for antibodies which agglutinate sheep red blood cells occasionally gives false-positive results and is less reliable in childhood. During the infection, antibodies to Epstein–Barr virus capsid antigen are produced: IgM antibody persists for a few months and IgG antibody indefinitely.

HIV

HIV, which is responsible for AIDS, has produced a worldwide epidemic. It is estimated that 10–13 million adults are now infected with HIV, and that some 2 million adults and 600000 children have AIDS.

Clinical manifestations of HIV range from asymptomatic to life-threatening, and the cutaneous manifestations are just as heterogeneous. Skin diseases rarely present typically in HIV-infected persons, and more often are atypical, more exuberant, more widespread, or more resistant to standard therapies. With this in mind, the clinician must have a high index of suspicion to recognize, diagnose and treat the multitude of skin diseases found in HIV-infected individuals.

Although much is known about the epidemiology, transmission and natural history of the infection, less is known about how its presence affects the efficacy of diagnostic tools that dermatologists have come to rely on.

PRIMARY HIV INFECTION

The earliest manifestation of an HIV infection may be seen as an acute illness associated with seroconversion. This was first described in 1984 when a nurse was infected by an accidental needlestick. A mononucleosis-like illness is most frequently described. Fever and a rash are most commonly found, and flu-like symptoms of sore throat, myalgia, lethargy, malaise and headache can be found in almost half of the patients.

Laboratory results are non-specific in this setting. Antigenaemia in symptomatic seroconversion has been detected in 44–75% of individuals. At this stage, the p24 core antigen can be measured in the serum, but the HIV antibody will not be positive for 1–2 months after the onset of symptoms. HIV can be cultured from blood or cerebrospinal fluid (CSF) at this time. Other laboratory findings such as lymphopenia, elevated erythrocyte sedimentation rate and CSF pleocytosis are non-specific, as are biopsies of skin lesions.

HIV-RELATED INFECTIONS

Syphilis

Since 1987 there has been a marked increase in the number of reported cases of syphilis. Studies have shown that syphilis and other ulcerative diseases of the genitals are more common in HIV-infected patients, and that these diseases increase the risk of acquiring and transmitting HIV.

Primary lues presents with a painless ulceration (chancre) about 21 days after inoculation. Chancres may appear in unusual areas such as the mouth, anus, axilla, and even glabrous skin, depending on the sexual practices of the individual. The best diagnostic test is still a dark-field examination, although there are non-pathogenic treponemas in the mouth which make such a test almost impossible to interpret if the primary lesion is in the oral cavity. *Treponema pallidum* is thin (0.25–0.3 μm) with 8–14 regular, tightly wound spirals and is 6–14 μm long. It rotates about the longitudinal axis with bending in the middle. Atypical spirochaetes are loosely coiled, thick and exhibit a writhing motion and frequent relaxation of coils. A single dark-field examination has a sensitivity of no more than 50%. Negative results may mean that insufficient number of organisms were present; the patient had already received antibiotics; the lesion was approaching natural resolution; or that the lesion was not syphilitic.

Serological tests, including rapid plasma reagin (RPR) and fluorescent treponemal-antibody absorption (FTA-Abs), may be positive in primary lues, even in HIV-infected individuals. Specific treponemal tests (FTA-Abs and microhaemagglutination assay for *Treponema pallidum* (MHA-TP)) become reactive earlier in the primary infection compared to the RPR or Venereal Disease Research Laboratory test (VDRL). The VDRL and RPR tests have similar sensitivities and specificities, but the RPR results can be read by the naked eye and are utilized by most routine laboratories (Table 6.1). The FTA-Abs is the most specific and most sensitive treponemal test but requires a fluorescence microscope, which is not always available. It becomes positive before MHA-TP in primary syphilis.

The serological manifestations of syphilis in the secondary and later stages are more controversial. Reports have described asymptomatic disease as well as more aggressive lues maligna, although a

Table 6.1   Sensitivity and specificity of serological tests

	Sensitivity (%)				Specificity (%)
	Primary	Secondary	Latent*	Late*	
VDRL	80 (74–87)	100	80 (71–100)	71 (37–94)	98
RPR-card	86 (81-100)	100	80 (53–100)	73 (36–96)	98
FTA-Abs	98 (93-100)	100	100	96	99
MHA-TP	82 (69-90)	100	100	94	99

*Widely variable results in the literature.

VDRL = Venereal Disease Research Laboratory; RPR-card = rapid plasma reagin-card; FTA-Abs = fluorescent treponemal-antibody absorption; MHA-TP = microhaemagglutination assay for *Treponema pallidum*.

large series of patients seen at a sexually transmitted disease (STD) clinic showed no significant differences in the clinical stage of syphilis or in the disease presentation when comparing HIV and non-HIV infected persons. Some investigators have found significantly higher serum RPR titres in HIV-infected individuals with secondary syphilis when compared with persons not infected with HIV. Likewise, there have been a few reports describing delayed or even absent serological reactivity in patients with proven syphilis.

In certain circumstances a negative RPR may simply represent the prozone effect where there is an antibody excess. Data from the early antibiotic era reported the prozone phenomenon in 1–2% of serum samples from patients with syphilis, although this figure may be higher in HIV infection, as HIV-infected persons may make more antibodies due to polyclonal B-cell activation. There is an optimal ratio of antigen to antibody which will reveal a visible soluble precipitate and thus a positive test. If there is excess antibody (prozone) or antigen (postzone), a false-negative test results (Fig. 6.1). This type of false-negative test can be rectified by diluting the patient's serum so that a more optimal concentration of antibody is present; however, most hospitals do not routinely test for the prozone phenomenon

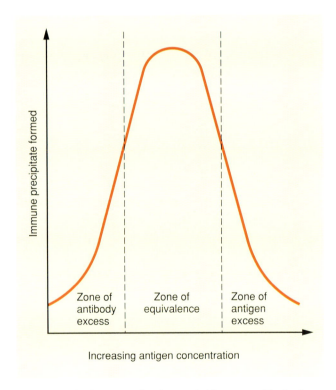

Fig. 6.1   Antigen–antibody precipitin curve. Typical precipitin curve resulting from titration of increasing antigen concentration plotted against amount of immune precipitate formed. Amount of antibody is kept constant throughout.

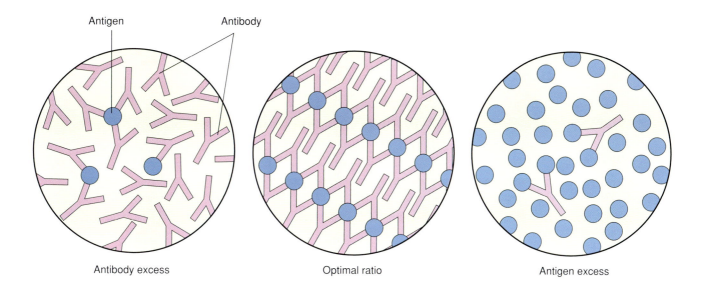

Antigen   Antibody

Antibody excess   Optimal ratio   Antigen excess

Fig. 6.2 The optimal ratio of antigen to antibody (middle) yields an insoluble precipitate in the classic precipitation test. The prozone phenomenon occurs in the situation depicted to the left (antibody excess). By diluting the specimen with antibody excess, the optimal antigen–antibody ratio will be obtained and the test will become positive.

and the physician may need to request that the serum be diluted (Fig. 6.2).

Normally the treponemal tests remain positive throughout life. In asymptomatic HIV-seropositive patients, 7% with a history of syphilis will lose reactivity to the treponemal tests. That figure increases to 38% of those with symptomatic HIV infection.

In general, the standard serological tests are accurate in the setting of AIDS, although when faced with negative serologies the clinician may need to perform skin biopsies to confirm lesions suspicious of lues. Plasma cell infiltration is a clue, but it may be absent or sparse in 25% of biopsy specimens. Silver stains are recommended in all suspected cases of secondary syphilis. Spirochaetes can be demonstrated in about a third of the cases, mainly around the superficial blood vessels and within the epidermis. Direct fluorescent antibody staining of lesion material can be done, and dark-field examinations should be performed.

Table 6.2 Forty-two reported cases of neurosyphilis in HIV-infected patients

Diagnosis	No. of patients
Asymptomatic neurosyphilis	5
Acute syphilitic meningitis	
Meningitis	9*
Cranial nerve dysfunction	15
Polyradiculopathy	1
Meningovascular syphilis	11
General paresis	1

*Five of these patients also had cranial nerve abnormalities.

There may be a shorter latency period for the development of neurosyphilis with HIV infection. It has not been well-documented at what point a lumbar puncture should be performed and what findings in the CSF are necessary to make the diagnosis of neurosyphilis. Asymptomatic cases of neurosyphilis have been documented, although most patients present with acute syphilitic meningitis or cranial nerve abnormalities (Table 6.2).

There are no CSF changes distinctive to syphilis, but at least one abnormality can be found in 97% cases in which a spinal tap is done

Table 6.3   Cerebrospinal fluid abnormalities in 42 reported cases of coexisting syphilis and AIDS

Abnormal value	Cells (%)	Protein (%)	Glucose (%)	VDRL (%)
Number with/total reported	29/34 (85)	28/34 (82)	11/32 (34)	31/39 (79)
Median	173	125	37	1:4
Range	8–2000	46–1000	11–42	wr 1:16

VDRL = Venereal Disease Reference Laboratory; wr = Weakly reactive.

(Table 6.3). The CSF VDRL, which is the gold standard, is negative in 21% of AIDS patients with proven neurosyphilis. Other abnormalities, such as pleocytosis, elevated levels of protein or changes in the glucose, can be detected in other diseases that affect the central nervous system. CSF pleocytosis and elevated protein or immunoglobulin levels have been reported in 30–69% of asymptomatic HIV-seropositive persons whose other serological tests showed no evidence of syphilis. A positive CSF VDRL is specific but a negative test does not rule out neurosyphilis. The diagnostic value of the FTA-Abs and MHA-TP in CSF analysis is unproven, but a non-reactive CSF specific treponemal test may be sufficient for exclusion of neurosyphilis.

At this time, standard diagnostic tools appear to be most useful in the AIDS population. Reaginic tests such as RPR and VDRL may not be as sensitive and the specific treponemal tests such as the FTA-Abs and MHA-TP may revert to negative in HIV infection, but overall appear to be reliable. Tests mainly used in research, such as PCR inoculation of rabbit testicles, *T. pallidum* haemagglutination index (TPHA), and others may become available in the future to help guide the clinician in such a protean disease.

Chancroid

Chancroid is a sexually transmitted infection characterized as acute painful ulcers on the genitalia accompanied by painful unilateral inguinal lymphadenopathy that can progress to suppurative buboes. Although possible with new solid-media culture techniques, culture of *Haemophilus ducreyi* is difficult due to its complex nutritional requirements, and most physicians do not have access to a laboratory capable of reliably growing these organisms. If available, specimens should be taken from the purulent ulcer base without extensive cleaning and kept at a temperature of 33°C in an environment of 1–5% carbon dioxide. Colonies appear in 2–4 days. Antimicrobial resistance has become more common and so testing for antibiotic sensitivity is recommended on all isolates.

A loop can be used to gather material from the undermined border of the lesion for direct examination. Some clinicians are able to identify the Gram-negative bacillus in the school-of-fish arrangement if stained with Unna-Pappenheim, Wright, Giemsa or Gram stains, but there are many false-positive and false-negative results. Electron microscopic examination has been recommended as a first-line test but most genital ulcers have a polymicrobial flora. Biopsies of the ulcer are not specific.

The Ito-Reenstierna skin test, once commonly used, is obsolete. Autoinoculation has many false-positive and false-negative results and is no longer recommended. Reliable serological tests are not yet available.

Gonorrhoea

Gonorrhoea is an STD which usually manifests as a urethritis or cervicitis. In general, there are no major modifications in the presentation or diagnosis in AIDS patients, although there are a few reports of unusual infections such as gonococcal osteomyelitis and even Fitz-Hugh and Curtis syndrome in a homosexual man. The diagnosis is made presumptively by the history, clinical findings and the presence of intracellular Gram-negative diplococci on Gram stain. Confirmation by culture of *Neisseria gonorrhoeae* is necessary. The reliability of culture is dependent on the number of sampling sites, techniques for collection, method and duration of transportation, growth medium, incubation conditions and the methods used for the identification of isolates. Cotton, dacron or calcium-alginate swabs may be used to collect specimens, but the use of antiseptics, analgesics and lubricants should be avoided.

Alternative methods have been looked at extensively, including enzyme-linked immunosorbent assay (ELISA) and immunofluorescence, DNA probes, genetic transformation and the limulus lysate assay, but offer no advantage in time or cost in symptomatic men or women.

Herpes infections

Members of the human herpesvirus family, including herpes simplex virus (HSV), varicella-zoster virus (VZV) and cytomegalovirus (CMV), are common pathogens in the immunocompromised host and represent a significant cause of morbidity and mortality. These double-stranded DNA viruses replicate within the nucleus, leading to cell death during acute infections, and then remain dormant in neuronal cells of ganglia, resulting in lifelong infection which under the appropriate circumstances can recrudesce.

HERPES SIMPLEX VIRUS (HSV)

Primary oral–facial herpes, usually caused by HSV-1, is predominantly a disease of children and young adults, with a variable clinical course. Diagnosis can be confirmed by culturing the virus from lesions, antigen detection, serum antibody assays, biopsy, Tzanck smears (as discussed in Chapter 2), or with the use of monoclonal antibodies and direct immunofluorescence.

Recurrent oral–facial herpes afflicts between 25 and 40% of the American population and more

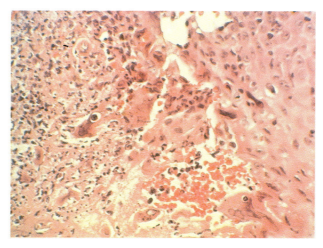

Fig. 6.3 Within a dense polymorphous inflammatory infiltrate, there are enlarged multinucleate giant cells typical of herpetic cytopathic change. Haematoxylin and eosin, × 200.

than 85% of the adult population throughout the world has serological evidence of HSV-1 exposure. The disease is usually milder and of shorter duration and can be triggered by exposure to sunlight, stress or, in the case of AIDS patients, the onset of a new opportunistic infection (Fig. 6.3). Diagnostic tools are the same, except that serum antibody testing is less helpful once a patient has a known clinical or virological history of HSV. These same principles apply for herpetic lesions at other cutaneous sites, including primary and recurrent genital herpes infections which are most commonly due to HSV-2.

In the USA, 16% of the population aged 15–74 has serological evidence of previous exposure to HSV-2 which is almost exclusively acquired sexually. The majority of these infections are clinically inapparent. In one study, 78% of women attending an STD clinic who had serological evidence of HSV-2 had no historical, clinical or virological evidence of genital herpes infection and 4% were asymptomatically shedding HSV. These infections especially are difficult to diagnose even in the immunocompetent population because the clinical signs and symptoms are so variable and, as previously mentioned, are not recognized by many patients. Cervical lesions may be visible or detectable only by colposcopy.

Serum antibodies to HSV-1 and HSV-2 are helpful initially to establish a diagnosis and for prognostic information since genital HSV-2 lesions are much more likely to recur. Viral cultures may be the most efficient means of confirming a clinical diagnosis with a first episode; however, obtaining samples from a single site has a sensitivity of less than 60%. Obtaining swabs from multiple anatomical sites including the anal area increases the sensitivity and all swabs can be placed in the same culture vial to maximize cost-effectiveness. Early first-episode ulcers yield positive viral cultures in up to 80% of patients but ulcers from recurrent infection are culture-negative in 50% of patients.

Although immunocompromised patients may have self-limited, localized disease, depending on the degree of immunosuppression, herpes infections may recur more frequently and have a more severe, prolonged course. Progressive, deep erosions and ulcerations may occur that persist for months with continuous shedding of HSV. This can occur even while the patient is on therapeutic or suppressive doses of acyclovir or foscarnet, confusing the clinical picture even further. It is especially important in these cases to try to culture the agent so that drug sensitivities can be performed.

VARICELLA-ZOSTER VIRUS (VZV)

Varicella, caused by the VZV, is also a disease usually seen in children, as evidenced by the high rates of VZV antibodies detected in the adult population. Like HSV, VZV establishes a latent infection in the sensory ganglia. Activation of VZV usually results in shingles, although haematogenous dissemination of virus from the affected ganglion can result in widespread cutaneous and visceral disease. Cellular immunity is more important than humoral immunity in the host's resistance to recurrent and reactivated VZV infections, which explains why patients with depleted T lymphocytes can suffer repeated attacks of herpes zoster. Indeed, the incidence of herpes zoster is greatly increased in patients with HIV and can be an early manifestation of HIV infection. As the HIV disease progresses, zoster can recur in different dermatomes and may persist chronically with unusual clinical manifestations ranging from verrucous or hyperkeratotic to ecthymatous lesions.

The diagnostic tests for varicella and herpes zoster are similar to HSV. Viral culture or the identification of viral antigens and nucleic acid from the lesions are the only reliable means of distinguishing VZV from HSV. Isolation of VZV from culture is much more difficult than HSV. Serum VZV antibody levels are needed to separate widespread herpes zoster from acute varicella. Tzanck smears (see Chapter 2) and biopsies can be done from the lesions to help establish the diagnosis of a herpesvirus infection, but cannot distinguish HSV from VZV. PCR is reliable and superior to viral culture in identifying VZV (Table 6.4).

Table 6.4 Comparison of Tzanck smears, cultures and polymerase chain reaction (PCR)

Clinical disease	Tzanck smear (%)	Viral culture (%)	PCR results* (%)	
			Stained*	Unstained
Herpes simplex virus	60	83	73	83
Varicella-zoster virus	75	44	88	97
Herpes simplex–varicella-zoster virus	68	63	81	90
Control patients	13	0	0	0

*Stained indicates PCR performed on stained Tzanck smear. Unstained preps were taken at the time of the Tzanck smear.

CYTOMEGALOVIRUS (CMV)

CMV is the commonest viral pathogen in patients with advanced AIDS. Retinitis and infection of the gastrointestinal tract are frequently encountered; however, dissemination is common as the immune system deteriorates. Cutaneous infection may develop from reactivation of a latent virus, by haematogenous spread, or autoinoculation in the periorificial areas by faecal, urinary or salivary shedding of the virus.

Specific skin lesions have not been characterized, although perianal ulcerations seem to be the most frequent cutaneous lesion of CMV. The diagnosis of cutaneous CMV can be difficult to establish (Fig. 6.4). Viral culture is not reliable and, when obtained from the perianal area, may simply represent viral shedding from the gastrointestinal tract and not true cutaneous infection.

Lesional biopsy may demonstrate the cytopathic changes of CMV. Immunohistochemical staining and DNA hybridization studies are helpful. PCR can be used to identify CMV. *In situ* studies, whether utilizing PCR or immunoperoxidase hybridization, are more valuable in confirming the pathogenic role of the virus and not just contamination.

EPSTEIN–BARR VIRUS

Epstein–Barr virus can result in oral hairy leukoplakia, and is fairly specific to HIV-related immunodeficiency (a few cases have been reported in iatrogenic immunosuppression). The diagnosis is relatively easy to make on clinical findings of a white corrugated lesion, most often located on the sides of the tongue. It does not rub off and can change from day to day. *Candida* must be excluded by a potassium hydroxide examination or with empirical antifungal therapy. Biopsy is helpful but not specific. Exfoliative cytology using the Papanicolaou stain has been shown to be a reliable and non-invasive way of diagnosing oral hairy leukoplakia. The smears demonstrate condensation and margination of the nuclear chromatin, described as nuclear beading. A definite diagnosis can be made by the demonstration of replicating Epstein–Barr virus in the keratinocytes by DNA *in situ* hybridization, immunohistochemistry or electron microscopy. Lesions which clinically and histologically look like oral hairy leukoplakia but do not contain Epstein–Barr virus have been termed pseudohairy leukoplakia.

Bacillary angiomatosis

Bacillary angiomatosis can present with dermal pyogenic granuloma-like lesions or subcutaneous skin-coloured or dusky nodules. *Rochalimaea henselae* and *R. quintana* have been identified as the causative agents. The bacilli are extremely difficult to culture and efforts to propagate the organism have failed. Culturing blood is enhanced with the use of lysis centrifugation and incubation using freshly prepared blood-enriched media; however, the efficiency of culture is unknown. Serological testing is not available and so, most often, the diagnosis depends on tissue biopsy (Fig. 6.5). Some or all of the following five histological features can be found:

- Epithelial collarettes.
- Lobular proliferation of small blood vessels

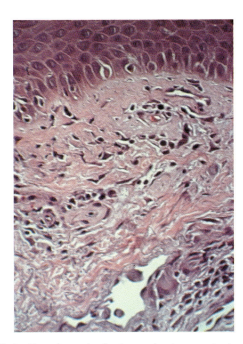

Fig. 6.4 Prominent inclusions of cytomegalovirus are found within endothelial cells in the papillary dermis in this human immunodeficiency virus-seropositive person. Haematoxylin and eosin, × 200.

lined by large, protuberant, cuboidal endothelial cells.

- Oedematous stroma.
- Polymorphonuclear leukocytes and neutrophilic debris.
- Eosinophilic granular clumps composed of clusters of bacteria.

The bacilli stain positively with Warthin-Starry silver stain, although this stain is non-specific. Electron microscopy can be used to confirm the diagnosis and shows clumps of pleomorphic bacilli with a Gram-negative trilaminar cell wall. PCR can be used to amplify and sequence ribosomal DNA from bacillary angiomatosis lesions, but this technique is not widely available to most clinicians.

Mycobacteria

The AIDS epidemic has led to a rapidly growing number of mycobacterial diseases, especially with *Mycobacterium tuberculosis* complex and *Mycobacterium avium-intracellulare* (MAI) complex (Fig. 6.6). There has also been a significant increase in infections due to typically non-pathogenic mycobacteria and other acid-fast organisms requiring special culture conditions. Communication between the clinician and the laboratory is especially crucial when these organisms are possible.

Tuberculosis of the skin is caused by *M. tuberculosis, M. bovis* or the bacillus Calmette-Guérin (BCG), which is an attenuated strain of *M. bovis*. Diagnosis may vary slightly depending on the host's immune response and the pattern of cutaneous disease present, i.e. scrofuloderma, lupus

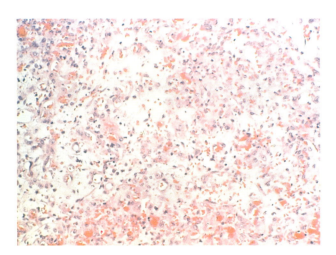

Fig. 6.5 Bacillary angiomatosis. There is a proliferation of vessels in an oedematous stroma. Focal haemorrhage and collections of neutrophils were present in the spaces between vessels. Haematoxylin and eosin, × 200.

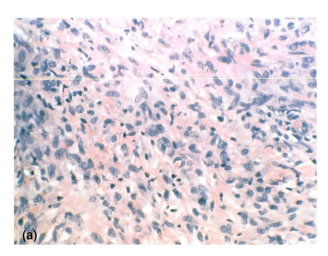

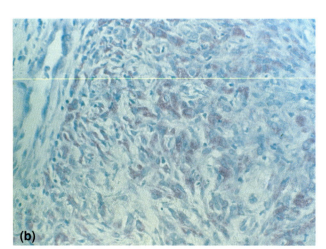

Fig. 6.6 Mycobacterial infections. (a) In the dermis, there is a dense infiltrate composed of mononuclear phagocytes, some of which are spindle-shaped.

(b) Special stains reveal myriads of acid-fast organisms. (a): Haematoxylin and eosin, × 400; (b) acid-fast, × 400.

vulgaris, tuberculosis verrucosa cutis. Tuberculin skin testing can be helpful if the patient is not anergic, as demonstrated by positive reactions to *Candida*, dermatophyte or other control skin tests. Biopsy of skin lesions for histological examination and for culture is crucial. Typical tubercles or acid-fast organisms may be absent. Smears and cultures of purulent drainage are valuable. New stains such as fluorescent auramine-rhodamine may improve the sensitivity since a greater amount of the clinical specimen can be examined with low-power microscopy.

Diagnosis of disease due to *M. ulcerans* is based on the presence of acid-fast bacilli in tissue sections and the microbial culture from a node or ulcer. *M. ulcerans* requires a lower temperature (30–32 °C) for growth. Skin testing with mycobacterial antigens is of no use. Healing of the lesions is always preceded by reversal of this anergic state.

M. haemophilum has been associated with cutaneous abscesses in AIDS patients, but can also cause bacteraemia. Direct acid-fast bacillus stains are usually positive. Histopathologically there is a mixed polymorphonuclear and granulomatous inflammation with no caseation necrosis. This organism requires iron-containing compounds, a lower temperature (30 °C) and up to 8 weeks of incubation.

Primary skin disease due to MAI complex is very rare, but cutaneous lesions may result from disseminated infection. Biopsies generally show non-caseating tuberculoid granulomas and acid-fast bacilli can be found: culture is necessary to confirm the diagnosis and to identify drug sensitivities. Blood cultures are particularly helpful as mycobacteraemia is probably continuous in AIDS patients.

Disease due to *M. kansasii is* endemic in Texas, Louisiana, Chicago, California and Japan and can occur in patients without immunosuppression. Histopathology is not helpful in differentiating it from tuberculosis, and skin testing is generally non-contributory. The diagnosis is confirmed by bacterial culture.

M. marinum can frequently be diagnosed clinically and biopsies of lesions usually show a tuber-culoid type of infiltrate. Confirmation requires culture of the bacterium which may grow better at 30 °C. The number of organisms present in a lesion may be very small and so lesions should be biopsied rather swabbed. PPD skin testing is not helpful.

A recently described mycobacterium *M. genavense,* has been detected in advanced HIV infection; most patients exhibit chronic fever, diarrhoea and weight loss. The organism appears only to grow in BATEC medium and more than 8 weeks may be required to detect growth.

M. fortuitum and *M. chelonae* may both cause disseminated infections in AIDS. Abscesses or a generalized maculopapular eruption has been described. Histopathology reveals necrosis, no caseation and acid-fast bacillus can sometimes be demonstrated in the microabscesses.

M. xenopi is an uncommon cause of disease, but can cause pulmonary or disseminated disease in AIDS patients. It is found more commonly in western Europe than in the USA. It grows more rapidly at 42 °C and so the laboratory should be notified if this organism is clinically suspected.

Traditional culture methods using Löwenstein–Jensen or Middlebrook media take 6 or more weeks of incubation. The new BATEC radiometric system and the Septi-Check acid-fast bacillus system to culture mycobacterium can shorten the average time to detection of growth by an average of 2 weeks. Advances such as new culture media have improved the ways laboratories identify and report results, but new methods of detecting mycobacteria directly from clinical specimens are needed. DNA probes currently available are not sensitive enough, as 10^5 to 10^6 organisms are required for detection. Newer techniques, such as PCR to amplify DNA, signal amplification targeted at RNA, and restriction fragment length polymorphism (RFLP), have been used to detect mycobacteria directly from clinical specimens. PCR is especially promising; however, the method is so sensitive that contamination of a laboratory with traces of the very stable segments of DNA could result in false-positive reactions.

Tuberculostearic acid (TSA), measured by gas–liquid chromatography, has been found to be a possible indicator of mycobacterial infection, but does not allow determination of the species. TSA is a structural component of the cell wall of all mycobacteria, corynebacteria, *Nocardia* and *Actinomyces*. In respiratory specimens, detection of TSA has a high degree of sensitivity and specificity, and its use may be even greater on CSF, which is normally sterile. ELISA has not shown a high enough sensitivity or specificity for routine use, and immunological techniques using catalase antigens are still being investigated. Even if these techniques are applied more routinely to the rapid diagnosis of mycobacterial diseases, routine procedures such as cultures will probably be necessary to follow drug sensitivities.

TROPICAL INFECTIONS

Leprosy

Mycobacterium leprae is an acid-fast bacillus that produces no known endotoxin or exotoxin. It can invade and multiply within peripheral nerves, endothelial and phagocytic cells. The immunological response of the host appears to be the main determinant of the clinical response to infection with *M. leprae*. The most widely used test to evaluate cell-mediated immunity is the Mitsuda or **lepromin skin test**. Heat-killed *M. leprae* is injected intradermally. Granulomatous reactions develop in persons who are capable of developing cell-mediated immunity to the bacillus. Positivity does not depend on previous exposure to the organism and is not a diagnostic test for leprosy. In fact, 50–90% of normal persons over the age of 5 years will have a positive test. Lepromatous patients with consistently negative skin tests during the course of their disease remain susceptible to reinfection or relapse after chemotherapy. Tests using other extracts of *M. leprae* have been used, but are not specific or diagnostic of leprosy either.

A test that is frequently relied on is the **bacterial index** (BI) and the **morphological test** (MI) determined from tissue smear. An incision of about 2–3 mm is made into a lesion. Fluid and cellular material is spread on a slide and stained with Ziehl–Neelsen carbolfuchsin. Counterstain with alkaline methylene blue is performed and the number of organisms are averaged from smears from the different lesions. Nasal scrapings can also be used, but expertise is required to differentiate *M. leprae* from non-pathogenic acid-fast bacilli found in any nose. The MI is used to evaluate treatment efficacy by correlating the number of viable bacilli with the number of solidly and uniformly staining bacteria. Intra- and interobserver variations can hinder the reliability of both the BI and MI.

Skin biopsies should include the dermis and panniculus. Bacilli are not usually found in tuberculoid forms but nerves are infiltrated and even replaced by granulomas. Borderline disease shows epithelioid granulomas and dermal nerves may show moderate swelling and infiltration. Acid-fast bacilli may sometimes be found. At the lepromatous pole, foamy macrophages predominate and acid-fast bacilli are invariably numerous.

Nerve biopsy may be necessary to confirm the diagnosis in pure neural leprosy. It is a special procedure which should be performed by experienced staff and in cases in which the diagnosis cannot otherwise be established. Sensory nerves such as the great auricular or the sural nerves should be sampled and only a few fasciculi should be taken.

The histamine test is used to diagnose postganglionic nerve injury. A pinprick is made over a drop of histamine diphosphate on lesional and non-lesional skin. A wheal can be observed at each site, but the red flare will not develop around the wheal if the intracutaneous nerve has been damaged. A methacholine sweat test is sometimes substituted in dark-skinned persons in whom a red flare may be difficult to detect. This tests for the absence of sweating in leprous lesions. The skin can also be tested for the presence or lack of tactile and temperature sensation.

Numerous tests utilizing phenolic glycolipid-1 (PGL-1) antigen have been studied. The measurement of antibodies to PGL-1 is of limited value for the diagnosis of leprosy as the positive and negative predictive values are low. Various serological assays have been applied, but again, are not very useful in the field. In general, the sensitivity of these tests are 80–100% for patients with multibacillary leprosy, and only 30–60% for patients with paucibacillary disease. Neopterin, a product of activated macrophages, may be a marker for reactional states, but prospective studies to establish the predictive value of the marker are lacking.

The most promising new technologies for diagnosing leprosy involve PCR and nucleic acid sequence-based amplification (NASBA). PCR has been reported by many researchers to be both sensitive and specific for detecting *M. leprae*. Thus far the test has little impact on the field diagnosis of disease except when signs are equivocal. It may become very important in the future to aid in the diagnosis of paucibacillary disease. One unique use thus far has been to show nasal carriage by healthy persons in an endemic community. Being able to identify sources of infection may lead to a better control of the disease. Little is known to date about the natural history of leprosy and HIV infection.

Leishmaniasis

Like leprosy, infection with the protozoan *Leishmania* can result in a wide spectrum of disease. Cutaneous (CL), mucocutaneous (MCL) and visceral (VL), diffuse cutaneous (DCL), kala-azar, post-kala-azar dermal leishmaniasis (PKDL), and leishmaniasis recidivans all present with unique clinical and diagnostic features. The clinical presentation of CL or VL in endemic areas will usually alert the physician to the diagnosis. It is in areas where leishmaniasis is rarely encountered that the diagnosis may be the most difficult. In experienced hands using multiple techniques, diagnosis can be confirmed (as defined by demonstration of the parasite) in roughly 70% of CL and 50% of MCL. In general, all the methods described below are more sensitive in lesions of less than 6 months' duration.

Cutaneous lesions can be aspirated, scraped or used for touch preps to set up smears and cultures. There seems to be no significant difference in yield between smears taken from the centre of an ulcer, ulcer border or from an incision made through intact skin at the margin of a lesion, although the slit smears may be slightly more sensitive. It should be remembered that tissue used for touch preps should not later be used for culture or histopathology, but can be used for DNA studies.

Once a smear is obtained, staining with Giemsa or Wright's is usually done. The amastigotes, which may be intracellular or extracellular, are only 2–4 μm, so oil microscopy is necessary. With Giemsa stain, the nucleus and kinetoplast are red-violet and the cytoplasm appears pale blue. Staining with fluorescein monoclonal antibodies directed against leishmanial antigens (genus- or species-directed) provides the most sensitive and specific way to identify amastigotes in a smear. These are not widely available but are used in research centres.

Histopathology can be the least sensitive diagnostic tool and results vary depending on differences in host immune response, the species and abundance of parasite, and the stage of disease when biopsied. Giemsa stain, immunofluorescence and immunoperoxidase staining of monoclonal antibodies to *Leishmania* can be used to enhance amastigote demonstration.

Culture of the organism is difficult and requires special media: usually a modified NNN (Nicolle–Novy–McNeal) is utilized. Antibiotics to inhibit bacterial growth are important, but antifungal agents will inhibit the growth of *Leishmania* and should be avoided. Cultures are maintained at 25–27 °C and may become positive as early as 1 week. They are more likely to be positive in cases where amastigotes can be demonstrated by direct examination. Hamsters are particularly susceptible to infection with *Leishmania*, and animal inoculation with tissue from a lesion can be performed. Diagnosis can be achieved within 2–12 weeks. Once cultured, species can be identified in a few specialized laboratories with isoenzyme electrophoresis, or monoclonal antibodies.

Serological assays are of little diagnostic use, especially in endemic areas. Most assays lack specificity and sensitivity, and cannot distinguish between leishmanial and trypanosomal infection.

Cross-reactions can also occur in malaria, toxo-plasmosis and amoebiasis. Humoral response is often lacking in patients with HIV and *Leishmania*. Immunofluorescent assays, direct agglutination tests, ELISA and complement fixation tests have all been employed.

The Montenegro **leishmanin skin test** can identify the presence of cell-mediated hypersensitivity to past or present infection. The test is considered positive if >5 mm induration is present. It may cross-react with *Trypanosoma* and *Leptomonas*. In addition, it is negative in active VL, PKDL, DCL and CL of less than 1 month's duration. Up to 15% of patients with CL and 4% of MCL patients may have a negative skin test.

DNA probes utilizing the kinetoplast DNA minicircles of *Leishmania* have been studied since the early 1980s. They are sensitive (detecting as few as 50 amastigotes) but are labour-intensive, and usually require radioactive detection systems. PCR allows for amplification of the target sequence, increasing the sensitivity (a single organism can be detected) to 87–100%. It is rapid and can be performed on biopsy tissue in the field. Contamination leading to false-positive results is the major drawback, but some investigators have adapted a method using DNase to help minimize this problem.

Coccidioidomycosis

Coccidioidomycosis is common in the south-western USA and other endemic areas of the western hemisphere. Most immunocompetent patients have a mild course, but immunocompromised individuals can have serious infections with haematogenous spread and recovery of *Coccidioides immitis* from blood cultures, inguinal lymph nodes and CSF.

This dimorphic fungus features spherules in tissue, but grows as a filamentous mould at room temperature with characteristic arthroconidia. It may take several weeks for these arthroconidia to appear and some saprophytic moulds possess arthroconidia as well, making confirmation tests necessary. Animal inoculations are time-consuming and exoantigen extractions are tech-nically difficult and expensive. Direct examination of purulent material from skin or sputum can sometimes reveal spherules suggestive of *C. immitis* when examined with calcofluor white or potassium hydroxide. Single endospores may be confused with phagocytic cells or other artefacts.

Serological tests have been a reliable means of establishing a presumptive diagnosis; however, the failure of these tests to detect coccidioidal antibodies does not exclude the diagnosis in immunocompromised patients or soon after infection in the immunocompetent. Circulating antigens cannot be reliably measured because the concentration of antigens appears to be low and they have not been fully characterized. ELISA procedures seem promising, but further studies are necessary better to define the sensitivity and specificity of this tool.

Like other infectious diseases in which the pathogen is slow or difficult to culture, tests utilizing DNA probes and PCR can be very useful. There is a commercially available DNA probe that targets specific rRNA sequences (Table 6.5). These probes are very specific and sensitive and can be used on clinical specimens or laboratory cultures.

Cryptococcosis

This is another disease which had been primarily an internal disease until the AIDS epidemic. Now cutaneous lesions are well-documented and clinically range from molluscum contagiosum-like to subcutaneous masses, draining sinuses, papules, pustules, plaques and cellulitis. It is the most common life-threatening fungal infection in HIV-infected patients.

Cryptococcus neoformans is a ubiquitous fungus which grows well at 30 and 37°C on all standard mycological media, although cyclohexamide will inhibit its growth. Skin lesions, pus, sputum, urine and CSF can be used as culture material. CSF or urine can be centrifuged, and the sediment prepared with Indian ink to help outline the capsule of *C. neoformans* which will appear as a halo around the budding yeast. Potassium hydroxide examination can be performed on sputum or pus. The small budding yeast with a narrow pore

Table 6.5   Pathogens with commercially available DNA probe detection assays

Bacteria	Fungi
Campylobacter spp. (CC)	*Blastomyces dermatitidis* (CC)
Chlamydia trachomatis (CC)	*Coccidioides immitis* (CC)
Enterococcus (CC)	*Cryptococcus neoformans* (CC)
Gardnerella vaginalis (CC)	*Histoplasma capsulatum* (CC)
Haemophilus influenzae (CC)	**Mycobacteria**
Legionella spp. (CC)	*Mycobacterium tuberculosis* (DS, CC)
Neisseria gonorrhoeae (DS, CC)	*Mycobacterium avium-intracellulare* (DS, CC)
Group A streptococcus (DS, CC)	*Mycobacterium gordonae* (CC)
Group B streptococcus (CC)	*Mycobacterium kansasii* (CC)
Streptococcus pneumoniae (CC)	**Viruses**
Staphylococcus aureus (CC)	Human papillomavirus (DS, IS)
Protoza	Cytomegalovirus (IS)
Trichomonas vaginalis (DS)	Epstein–Barr virus (IS)

CC = Culture confirmation assays; DS = direct specimen assays; IS = *in situ* hybridization assays.

between the mother and daughter cell must not be confused with cellular debris or leukocytes.

There are two patterns on histological examination of skin biopsies: either gelatinous or granulomatous (Fig. 6.7). The gelatinous pattern is characterized by numerous organisms with little or no tissue reaction. Granulomatous lesions show marked tissue reaction and even necrosis with a much smaller number of organisms. The capsule will not stain with haematoxylin and eosin or periodic acid–Schiff, but stains metachromatically purple with methylene blue, blue with alcian blue, or red with mucicarmine. The organism will stain black with the Fontana-Masson stain. Using a combination of Fontana-Masson and mucicarmine can be particularly useful in differentiating *C. neoformans* from *Blastomyces dermatitidis*.

Latex agglutination tests can be performed on CSF or serum, and are simple and fast. The specificity is high and more sensitive than the Indian ink preparation. The latex agglutination test can detect up to 93% of culturally proven cases, and can be invaluable in culture-negative cases. A single titre of 4 or less in serum or CSF is highly suggestive of cryptococcal infection, while a titre of 8 or more is indicative of active cryptococcosis. False-negative reactions are uncommon and have been attributed to the prozone phenomenon. False-positive reactions have been associated with rheumatoid factor (Table 6.6). The latex agglutination test has prognostic value. An increase in antigen titres usually indicates progressive disease, while failure of the titre to fall during therapy implies inadequate therapy.

Histoplasmosis

Disease caused by the dimorphic fungus, *Histoplasma capsulatum*, is endemic in the Ohio and Mississippi river valleys in the USA, the Caribbean, Central and South America and Africa. Disseminated histoplasmosis in AIDS patients may be rapidly fulminant, making early diagnosis paramount.

Cultures of blood and bone marrow are

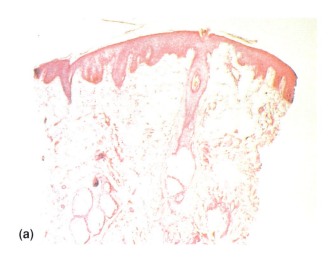

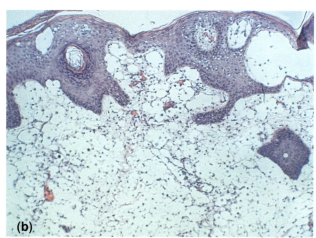

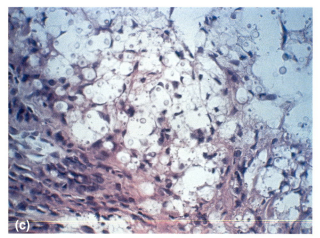

Fig. 6.7 Cryptococcosis. (a) In the superficial dermis, there is pale staining. (b) Higher magnification reveals small organisms embedded in a pale-staining matrix. (c) This magnification clearly reveals organisms, confirmed by culture to be *Cryptococcus*, in a pale-staining stroma. Haematoxylin and eosin; (a) × 40, (b) × 200, (c) × 400.

Table 6.6 False-positive cryptococcal latex agglutination tests

Rheumatoid factor

Trichosporon beigelii

DF2

Klebsiella pneumoniae

positive in 83% and 71% respectively of documented cases in patients with AIDS. Standard mycological culture media can be used but growth may not be detected for 2–4 weeks. Lysis-centrifugation techniques can decrease the recovery time to an average of 13 days. As with other dimorphic fungi, exoantigen studies can be performed on aqueous extracts of mature cultures and are especially useful to help identify atypical forms of the microorganism. Reference antisera are not routinely available, however.

Giemsa or Wright's stain can be used for the direct examination of sputum, bronchial specimens, urine, peripheral blood, bone marrow, CSF, pus or material taken from ulcers (Fig. 6.8). A presumptive identification can be made when 2–4 μm organisms are seen extracellulary or intracellularly within monocytes or macrophages (Fig. 6.8). The organism is composed of deeply stained protoplasm at one end of the cell and a large clear vacuole. Although this can be performed quickly, typical organisms are not always found, ranging from 12% of cases in blood to 75% in bone marrow.

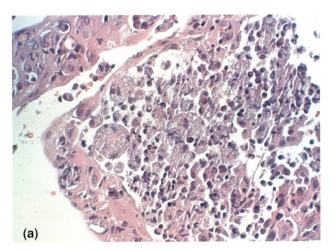

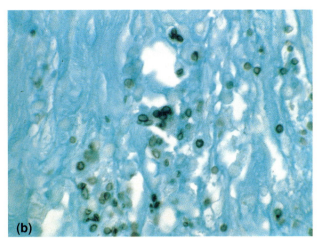

Fig. 6.8 (a) *Histoplasma* are revealed as pale-staining inclusions within the cytoplasm of mononuclear phagocytes. (b) Special stains more clearly reveal these fungal forms. (a) Haematoxylin and eosin, × 200; (b) Gomori methenamine silver, × 400.

Standard serological tests have a high incidence of false-positive and false-negative results in AIDS patients with disseminated disease. Solid-phase radioimmunoassay to detect a *H. capsulatum* polysaccharide antigen (HPA) can be used to help establish a diagnosis, as HPA can be found in high levels in urine (97%) and blood (79%) in AIDS patients. It is particularly useful in diagnosing relapses. An increase by 2 or more radioimmunoassay units of the HPA measured from the blood or urine strongly suggests relapse in AIDS patients and can be detected even before clinical relapse is suspected. Complement fixation tests are less accurate and may even be negative in immunosuppressed patients.

Onchocerciasis

Onchocerca volvulus is a nematode estimated to infect 18 million people in Africa, Central and South America, Saudi Arabia and Yemen. Identification of the adult parasite can be made on biopsy of nodules (Fig 6.9) which are characteristically located over bony prominences. Ultrasonography may be used to help identify occult nodules. Superficial **skin snips** can be taken from the scapula, iliac or thigh area and placed on a glass slide with normal saline (Fig.

6.10). A coverslip is applied and, under the microscope, microfilaria can be seen wriggling out at the edges of the skin.

The Mazzotti test involves the oral administration of 50 mg of diethylcarbamazine. A positive reaction consists of oedema, fever, arthralgia and an exacerbation of pruritus. Its use is no longer recommended for the routine diagnosis of onchocerciasis as it can exacerbate ocular disease.

The development of serodiagnostic assays has been hampered by the immunological cross-reactivity among nematodes. Preliminary work with different antigens is promising and may soon result in a serological assay that is available to the clinician. PCR can improve the detection of patients, even in those with microfilaria-negative skin snips, although this tool is not readily available (Table 6.7).

Trichinosis

Ingestion of *Trichinella spiralis* larva-containing cysts, usually in inadequately cooked pork, may cause trichinosis. Diagnosis can be confirmed by demonstrating larvae in striated muscle. The muscle biopsy should be large and, even then, trichinae cannot usually be found unless the infection is very heavy and of more than 1

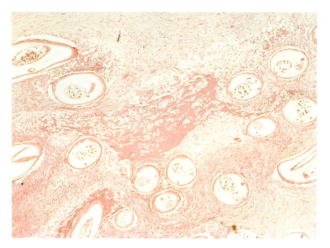

Fig. 6.9 Adult *Onchocerca volvulus* in nodule of soft tissue. Haematoxylin and eosin, × 200.

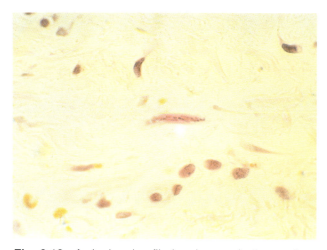

Fig. 6.10 A single microfilarium is seen in the papillary dermis of skin. Haematoxylin and eosin, × 300.

Table 6.7 Infectious pathogens detected by polymerase chain reaction associated with cutaneous disorders

Viruses
  Herpes simplex virus
  Cytomegalovirus
  HTLV I + HTLV-II
  HIV-1 + HIV-2
  Epstein–Barr virus
  Human papillomavirus
  Measles
  Adenovirus
  Parvovirus
  Varicella-zoster virus

Bacteria
  Mycobacterium tuberculosis
  Mycobacterium avium
  Mycobacterium leprae
  Neisseria gonorrhoeae
  Borrelia burgdorferi
  Chlamydia
  Treponema pallidum
  Rochalimaea henselae
  Rochalimaea quintana

Fungi
  Blastomyces dermatitidis
  Coccidioides immitis
  Cryptococcus neoformans
  Histoplasma capsulatum

Parasites
  Trypanosoma
  Leishmania
  Toxoplasma
  Schistosoma
  Onchocerca volvulus

HTLV = Human T-cell lymphotrophic virus; HIV = human immunodeficiency virus.

month's duration. Eosinophilia is present in 80% of cases but is not specific. Immunofluorescence antibody tests and the bentonite flocculation test are useful in establishing a diagnosis. An intradermal skin test can give a response within 15 min but usually does not become positive before the third week of infection.

Serological assays are being developed. An IgG-ELISA using an excretory-secretory antigen has shown 100% specificity but is not reliably positive if tested earlier than day 23 or later than day 700 of the infection.

FURTHER READING

Beard J, Benson P, Skillman L. Rapid diagnosis of coccidioidomycosis with a DNA probe to ribosomal RNA. *Archives of Dermatology* 1993; **129**: 1589–1593.

Cotell S, Noskin G. Bacillary angiomatosis. Clinical and histologic features, diagnosis and treatment. *Archives of Internal Medicine* 1994; **154**: 524–528.

Crumpacker C, Gulick R. Herpes simplex. In: Fitzpatrick T, Eisen A, Wolff K, Freedberg I, Austen K (eds) *Dermatology in General Medicine*, 4th edn. McGraw-Hill, New York, 1993, pp. 2531–2543.

Garcia-Patos V, Pujol R, Curell R, de Moragas J. Cytomegalovirus-induced cytopathic changes in skin biopsies specimens: clinicopathologic study in patients with the acquired immunodeficiency syndrome and an active extracutaneous cytomegalovirus infection. *Archives of Dermatology* 1992; **128**: 1552–1553.

Hook E, Marra C. Acquired syphilis in adults. *New England Journal of Medicine* 1992; **326**: 1060–1069.

Ison C. Laboratory methods in genitourinary medicine. Methods of diagnosing gonorrhoea. *Genitourinary Medicine* 1990; **66**: 453–459.

Jurado R, Campbell J, Martin P. Prozone phenomenon in secondary syphilis: has its time arrived? *Archives of Internal Medicine* 1993; **153**: 2496–2498.

Kalter D. Laboratory tests for the diagnosis and evaluation of leishmaniasis. *Dermatologic Clinics* 1994; **12**: 37–50.

Kinloch-de Loes S, de Saussure P, Saurat J, Stalder H, Hirschel B, Peerin L. Symptomatic primary infection due to human immunodeficiency virus type I: review of 31 cases. *Clinical Infectious Diseases* 1993; **17**: 59–65.

Kiehn T. The diagnostic mycobacteriology laboratory of the 1990s. *Clinical Infectious Diseases* 1993; **17** (suppl 2): S447–S454.

Kirchner J. Resurgence of syphilis. *Infections in Medicine* 1994; **11**: 292–296, 307.

Klaster P. Laboratory techniques for diagnosis. *Tropical and Geographical Medicine* 1944; **46**: 58–60.

Klaster P. Serology of leprosy. *Tropical and Geographical Medicine* 1994; **46**: 115–118.

LeBoit P, Berger T, Egbert B, Beckstead J, Yen T, Stoler M. Bacillary angiomatosis, the histopathology and differential diagnosis of a pseudoneoplastic infection in patients with human immunodeficiency virus disease. *American Journal of Surgery and Pathology* 1989; **13**: 909–920.

Leichsenring M, Troger J, Nelle M, Buttner D, Darge K, Doehring-Schwerdtfeger E. Ultrasonographical investigations of onchocerciasis in Liberia. *American Journal of Tropical Medicine and Hygiene* 1990; **43**: 380–385.

Lopez M, Inga R, Cangalaya M *et al*. Diagnosis of *Leishmania* using the polymerase chain reaction: a simplified procedure for field work. *American Journal of Tropical Medicine and Hygiene* 1993; **49**: 348–356.

Mahannop P, Chaicumpa W, Setasuban P, Morakote N, Tapchaisri P. Immunodiagnosis of human trichinellosis using excretory-secretory (ES) antigen. *Journal of Helminthology* 1992; **66**: 297–304.

Musher D. Syphilis, neurosyphilis, penicillin, and AIDS. *Journal of Infectious Diseases* 1991; **163**: 1201–1206.

Myers S, Prose N, Bartlett J. Progress in the understanding of HIV infection: an overview. *Journal of the American Academy of Dermatology* 1993; **29**: 1–21.

Nahass G, Goldstein B, Zhu W, Serfling U, Penneys N, Leonardi C. Comparison of Tzanck smear, viral culture, and DNA diagnostic methods in detection of herpes simplex and varicella-zoster infection. *Journal of the American Medical Association* 1992; **268**: 2541–2544.

Ogunrinade A, Chandrashekar R, Eberhard M, Weil G. Preliminary evaluation of recombinant *Onchocerca volvulus* antigens for serodiagnosis of onchocerciasis. *Journal of Clinical Microbiology* 1993; **31**: 1741–1745.

Pedersen C, Lindhardt B, Jensen B. Clinical course of primary HIV infection: consequences for subsequent course of infection. *British Medical Journal* 1989; **299**: 154–157.

Warren R, Perceval A, Dwyer B. Comparative evaluation of cryptococcal latex tests. *Pathology* 1993; **25**: 76–80.

Zarabi C, Thomas R, Adesokan A. Diagnosis of systemic histoplasmosis in patients with AIDS. *Southern Medical Journal* 1992; **85**: 1171–1175.

Chapter 7

Investigation of hair disorders

Rodney P. R. Dawber

■ **Hair growth**

■ **Hair and hair follicle microscopy**
Optical microscopy
Electron microscopy
Follicular microscopy

■ **Assessment of hirsutism and androgenetic alopecia**
Clinical assessment
Laboratory tests available
    Total testosterone (TT)
    Free testosterone (FT)
    Dehydroepiandrosterone sulphate
        (DHEA-S)
    Dihydrotestosterone (DHT)
    Androstenedione
    Sex hormone-binding globulin (SHBG)
    3α–Androstandiol glucuronide
        (3α–adiol G)
    Luteinizing hormone/follicle-stimulating
        hormone (LH/FSH)
Endocrine investigations related to clinical
    presentations

■ **Hair growth methodology**
Length of the hair cycle: examination of
hair roots
    Histological techniques
    Follicle kinetics
Hair shaft length and diameter
measurements
Compound measurements
    Hair pluckability
Growth pattern analysis

HAIR GROWTH

This chapter will consider methods of studying hair growth and also microscopic methods for detailed examination of hair shafts and hair follicles. In addition, the principles of the clinical and laboratory assessment of endocrine faults in hair growth are considered.

Hair growth proceeds through three distinct phases: a prolonged growth or **anagen** phase, a short involutional or **catagen** phase, and a final resting or **telogen** phase. About 90% of a person's scalp hair is in a continual growth phase which lasts between 2 and 6 years. Ten per cent of the scalp hair is in the telogen phase, which lasts between 2 and 3 months. At the end of the telogen phase, the hair is shed. Shedding 50–100 hairs a day is considered normal. When hair is shed, it is replaced by new hair from the same hair follicle. No new follicles are formed during one's life. Scalp hair grows about 1 cm a month. With age the rate of new hair growth diminishes, resulting in gradual thinning.

History-taking is of fundamental importance in assessing hair loss, which may be **localized** (as is usual in alopecia areata) or **diffuse**. The causes of alopecia are shown in Table 7.1. A patient with alopecia areata does not require extensive investigation and an autoantibody screen is not essential to the clinical management. Increased hair loss may occur after childbirth or after an acute illness such as an infection, when the problem usually lasts a few months and is self-limiting. It is necessary to take a careful history regarding the ingestion of drugs, including cancer chemotherapy agents, anticoagulants and retinoids. Treatable causes of diffuse hair loss include iron-deficiency anaemia and hyper- or hypothyroidism (see Chapter 3).

A patient complaining of balding or hair loss may, in fact, have an increased shedding rate or a decrease in hairs per unit area. The complaint of thinning of the hair may be due to a decrease in the number of hairs per unit or a decrease in hair diameter; sometimes this may be worsened by a decrease in hair pigmentation. By careful questioning, it is possible to assess the factors which guide one into particular lines of investigation and differential diagnosis. It is important to quantify these factors in order to assess accurately the progress of hair disease and also to assess the changes induced by treatment. For example, in androgenetic alopecia and hirsutism, changes in the telogen count, linear growth rate, diameter of hair and pigmentation are detectable before the affected individual is able subjectively to observe the changes.

Hair growth may be assessed by several simple clinical investigations. Daily hair growth may be measured with a graduated rule after shaving the skin. The length of the growth cycle (anagen) may be calculated by dividing the overall length of an uncut hair by the daily growth rate. In some circumstances it is only necessary to know the relative proportion of telogen/anagen hairs; this may be assessed by plucking hairs to examine the

Table 7.1 The causes of alopecia
Alopecia areata
Scarring alopecia
Discoid lupus erythematosus
Lichen planus
Pseudopelade
Hair loss in systematic disease
Telogen effluvium (e.g. after an acute illness or major surgery)
Iron-deficiency anaemia
Hyper- or hypothyroidism
Drug-induced alopecia (e.g. cancer chemotherapy agents)
Androgenetic alopecia
Traumatic alopecia
Trichotillamania
Related to hairstyle
Congenital alopecia
Monilethrix (beaded hair)
Pili torti (twisting)
Trichorrhexis nodosa (nodal fracture and fragility of hair)
Pili annulati (banded hair)

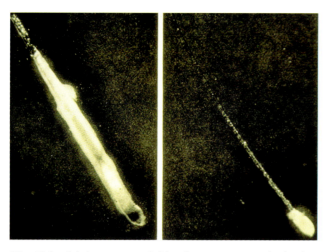

Fig. 7.1 (a) Anagen and (b) telogen roots – plucked hairs (light micrograph).

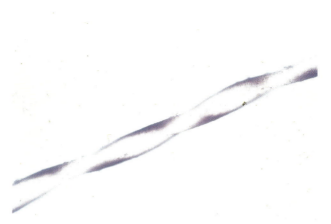

Fig. 7.2 Hair shaft showing pili torti, dry mounted; much 'glare' and lack of detail, but diagnosis is obvious (cf. Fig. 7.4, scanning electron micrograph).

roots or by skin biopsy (Fig. 7.1). It should be noted that, in general, only telogen hairs are removed by combing or washing. Detailed methods for assessing hair growth, as used in specialist departments, are discussed subsequently.

HAIR AND HAIR FOLLICLE MICROSCOPY

Hair shaft microscopy is essential for the diagnosis of many abnormalities, particularly fungal disease, congenital and hereditary hair shaft disorders, and to assess hair weathering.

In the diagnosis of fungal diseases of hair, plucked hairs are mounted in 20% aqueous potassium hydroxide solution; if the microscopy is to be carried out within 30 min then the addition of dimethylsulphoxide 40% (DMSO) may speed the clearing time. DMSO may cause false-negative results beyond this time since hyphal destruction occurs. The kerion type of infection may show only arthrospores on the proximal part of the plucked hair shaft despite massive inflammatory changes in the skin.

Optical microscopy

Routine light microscopy of hair shafts is essential for the diagnosis of diseases such as hereditary and congenital shaft abnormalities. To assess intrinsic shaft changes, only the proximal 1–2 cm of plucked hairs should be examined since more distal changes may be extrinsic and due to weathering. Hairs may be mounted dry if they are required for further studies; however, in routine transmitted light microscopic examination, the surface of dry-mounted hairs will scatter light (Fig. 7.2). More detail is seen and higher magnification will be possible if a standard mounting medium is used; potassium hydroxide and water are not satisfactory.

'Colour' changes seen by routine light microscopy may be due to pigment alterations, or structural changes not transmitting light and thus giving dark areas. If reflected light is used then the dark areas in structural diseases such as pili annulati become light; pigmentation changes are not altered by this technique. Careful examination using routine light microscopy provides most of the information required in clinical practice.

Polarization microscopy may provide extra information regarding the biochemical make-up of the hair and fine structural changes may become more obvious. Using this method it is possible to determine refractive index and the birefringence of fibres (the numerical difference between the refractive indices parallel and perpendicular to the hair axis), a physical phenomenon that reflects the orientation of internal structures in the hair. In the examination of hair from patients with the trichothiodystrophy symptom complex, polarizing microscopy reveals striking bright and dark regions on viewing the hair between cross-polarizers. Turning the microscopic stage approximately 10° (5° on each side of the position of maximum extinction) reverses the bright and dark areas: between cross-polarizers with the hair axis parallel to the vibration direction of the polarizer (maximum extinction or 0°), the hair reveals lines – tiger tail or zig zag hairs. This abnormality is associated with sulphur and high sulphur (matrix) protein deficiency.

The subtlety of optical microscopic methods can be enhanced by various specialized techniques. The scale pattern can be analysed in detail by examining a hair cast or impression of the hair in a suitable plastic material; an impression made by rolling the hair in the medium enables the whole circumference to be viewed. Interference microscopy, using monochromatic sodium light, greatly facilitates the examination of minute surface changes.

Electron microscopy

Optical microscopy is limited in resolution to approximately 0.2 mm and has a narrow depth of focus. Transmission electron microscopy is capable of very high resolution (down to 2 nm for biological materials) and has a depth-of-image focus that is greater than the normal specimen thickness (approximately 100 nm). Routine electron microscopic preparation may be suitable for examination of hair follicles, but the presence of keratinized hair within the follicle and the nature of hair structure make it necessary to modify a routine procedure to get the best resolution and

meaningful results. Glass knives give poor sectioning: a diamond knife is necessary for cutting ultrathin sections of hair without distortion. Needless to say, this is a very skilful procedure which is not always available in electron microscope laboratories.

Hair displays a homogeneous electron density and must be stained with a heavy metal to show anatomical detail. Uranyl acetate and lead citrate enable the overall structure to be seen; dodeca-tungstophosphoric acid gives added detail of cortex matrix proteins and cortical cell membranes. For transverse sections of hair fibres, ammoniacal silver or the silver methenamine stain which specifically stain cystine give more contrast to cuticular and cortical structure (Fig. 7.3) by highlighting the cystine-rich exocuticle and cortical matrix protein.

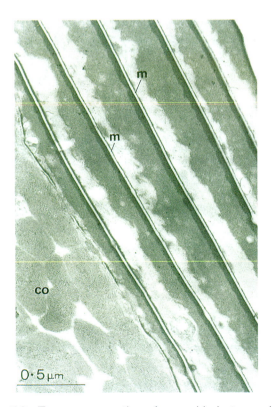

Fig. 7.3 Transverse section of normal hair–transmission electron micrograph, silver methenamine stain. The darker the colour, the greater the density of high sulphur protein. co = Cortex; M = cuticular cell membrane.

Scanning electron microscopy is very diverse in its modes of operation and gives a wealth of information about surface architecture (Fig. 7.4) elemental composition (if an X-ray microanalytical attachment is available), crystalline make-up and electrical and magnetic properties of specimens. It is a research tool and it cannot be stressed too greatly that all the detail needed by the clinician regarding hair microstructure can be obtained by optical microscopic methods.

Follicular microscopy

Biopsy technique must be carefully considered if useful histological results are to be obtained. The level of the biopsy must extend deep into subcutaneous fat to avoid cutting off hair bulbs. The epidermal surface of the excised tissue should be

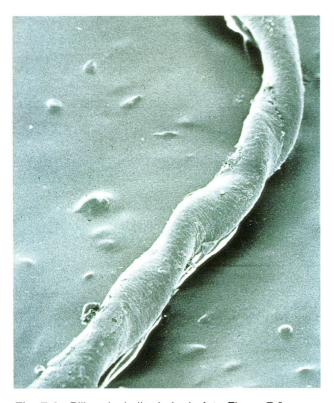

Fig. 7.4 Pili torti: similar hair shaft to Figure 7.2 (scanning electron micrograph).

apposed to a rigid piece of paper, to avoid curling of the tissue, and immediately placed in fixative; if necessary, it can be glued or pinned to the paper if longitudinal follicular cutting is desired, since follicles have a great propensity for bending prior to hardening, leading to cross-cutting in the dermis. Punch biopsies (6 mm) and horizontal sectioning at various levels give more dynamic information about the hair cycle status at the site from which the tissue was taken.

After processing, the embedded tissue requires careful orientation before cutting to maximize the chance of obtaining longitudinal follicular sections. Routine paraffin-embedded tissue has never been entirely satisfactory for visualizing cytological detail within the follicle; where possible, tissue should be fixed and embedded as for routine microscopy and 1 mm sections cut to give greater cytological clarity. Haematoxylin and eosin staining reveals the general detail of the various cell layers in the follicle.

Other histochemical stains may specifically enhance the appearance of various cell layers. The lower border of the internal root sheath takes up the Giemsa stain; this stains the keratinized internal root sheath specifically dark blue. The intrafollicular hair cuticle stains with toluidine blue and rhodamine B, first becoming visible as a thin blue layer surrounding the presumptive hair. The Van Gieson stain gives a yellow colour to the hair and the club in telogen roots; the tissue surrounding the club is brownish-red with PASHPA stain, whilst rhodamine B stains the cuticle a faint blue colour and the surrounding tricholemmal layer brilliant red.

Useful screening techniques for abnormal hair keratins are the fluorescence methods using either acridine orange or thioflavine T: normal hair keratin fluoresces blue with dilute acridine orange, whereas altered keratins such as the tip of hairs in trichorrhexis nodosa, dystrophic hairs in kwashiorkor, or weathered fibres fluoresce red or orange. The peracetic oxidation and thioflavine I fluorescent method stain the disulphide bonds in cystine, enabling sites of mature keratin to be detected in the exocuticle or cortex – SH bonds can be specifically stained by a fluorogenic maleimide N(7-dimethyl-amino-methyl coumarinyl) maleimide (DACM). This substance only fluoresces on combining with -SH bonds. This method requires frozen tissue; it has the advantage that the emission maximum of DACM does not overlap with any of the aromatic residues of proteins such as tryptophan. Many keratin-specific methods now exist for defining epidermal root sheath and matrix keratins – these need more assessment to define potential uses in clinical practice.

ASSESSMENT OF HIRSUTISM AND ANDROGENETIC ALOPECIA

Clinical assessment

Very careful clinical history, and general examination should be undertaken if hirsutism or androgenetic alopecia is the presenting sign. If no other virilizing symptoms or signs are found clinically, most authorities would accept this as normal or idiopathic or cryptogenic and therefore not carry out laboratory studies. The clinical severity of hirsutism can be numerically assessed. Androgenetic alopecia is graded by pattern definition – either the Ludwig diffuse forms (grades 1–3; Fig. 7.5) or the Hamilton grades 1–8 of the more typically male patterns (Fig. 7.6). Note that after the menopause (in some studies) up to 37% of normal women have demonstrated subtle forms of the male patterning – in endocrine terms, the sexes overlap.

A practical guide to the investigation of hirsutism is given in Chapter 3. However, in some medical cultures database laboratory studies are the norm for any sign or signs of potential androgen excess, no matter how mild the clinical appearance. In view of this, and the fact that some or all of the tests will be necessary in the more severe clinical presentations, one must consider the nature and potential value of each hormonal assay by outlining the tests available and their significance if abnormal, and the investigations to be carried out related to the clinical presenting signs.

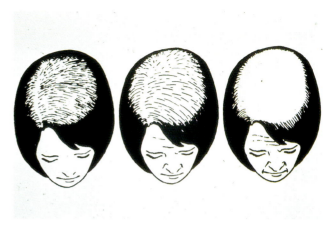

Fig. 7.5 Ludwig patterns of androgenetic alopecia, most common in females.

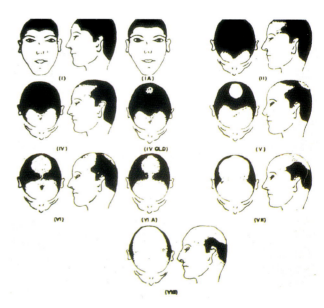

Fig. 7.6 Hamilton patterns of androgenetic alopecia, most common in males.

It is very important to relate the results to carefully compiled reference measurement which may vary to some degree from laboratory to laboratory; in this regard, whether the patient is pre-, peri- or post-menopausal is important, as is the stage of the menstrual cycle when the blood or urine was collected.

Laboratory tests available

TOTAL TESTOSTERONE (TT)

Normal values are <1.1 ng/ml. If the result is >2.0 ng/ml, it is mandatory to consider extensive studies of the adrenal glands and the ovaries, in particular regarding a possible androgen-secreting tumour. With borderline results, some authorities suggest measuring the mean of three separate TT results.

FREE TESTOSTERONE (FT)

This is a more sensitive indicator of hyperandrogenism than TT but it is more expensive to carry out and not routinely necessary. It may be useful in the monitoring of treatment using ovarian suppression.

DEHYDROEPIANDROSTERONE SULPHATE (DHEA-S)

Some authorities consider this to be the most frequently abnormal test in idiopathic hirsutism and androgenetic alopecia. High levels of DHEA-S have been reported, even in men with androgenetic alopecia. Levels over 700 mg/dl suggest an androgen-secreting tumour.

DIHYDROTESTOSTERONE (DHT)

This reflects mixed sites of origin in the ovaries, adrenals and peripheral conversion from testosterone. It is sometimes used as an arbitrator of normality or disease when TT, DHEA-S and cortisol are normal.

ANDROSTENEDIONE

This is usually elevated in hyperandrogenism but not in isolation. Note that any but the most recent published studies using this measure should probably be disregarded because of cross-reactivity with testosterone.

SEX HORMONE-BINDING GLOBULIN (SHBG)

This assay is very non-specific, being depressed when circulating androgens are raised; and SHBG is raised by oestrogens. It is often used in evaluating the ratio of testosterone to SHBG – it is more discriminating than T or SHBG alone.

3α-ANDROSTANDIOL GLUCURONIDE (3α-ADIOL G)

This remains an investigative tool until more detailed studies have been carried out; it is expensive. Being a DHT metabolite, it is used as an indicator of peripheral androgen action, reflecting 5α-reductase activity. Androsterone glucuronide (Adiol-G) is said to be more sensitive, although it is of uncertain value in clinical practice.

In clinical states suggesting that cortisol faults may exist, for example, congenital adrenal hyperplasia, the skills, judgement and facilities of the endocrinologist may be better employed. 17α-Hydroxyprogesterone, 11-deoxycortisol, the adrenocorticotrophic hormone stimulation test, the dexamethasone suppression test and the nafarelin stimulation test may all have a place in diagnosis and differential diagnosis – the reader is referred to more detailed endocrine texts for further discussion of these.

LUTEINIZING HORMONE/FOLLICLE STIMULATING HORMONE (LH/FSH)

These are widely used in clinical practice, often quite uncritically. They are often used when chronic anovulation exists and are commonly used to aid in the diagnosis of polycystic ovary disease (PCOD). Serum LH may be useful in corroborating the diagnosis of PCOD; however, it is not entirely specific to this disease and is occasionally normal in proven cases of PCOD.

Endocrine investigations related to clinical presentations

The presence of a single androgen-driven skin sign such as hirsutism or androgenetic alopecia alone does not necessarily constitute evidence of systemic virilization or a hormone-secreting lesion. It is therefore difficult to provide exact guidelines on the tests to perform in relation to the presenting signs, particularly since from country to country the needs and actions of differing social and medical cultures may vary the routine laboratory database required in conditions such as hirsutism or androgenetic alopecia.

The brief guidelines that follow are therefore attempting to defer to a 'middle-of-the-road' approach.

One can conveniently divide the clinical presentations into four groups:

- Mild hirsutism, often evolving only slowly over many years: the patient may only have concerns about the hair at one site, e.g. the chin. Ludwig-pattern alopecia grade 2 or less in any age group; Hamilton pattern alopecia grade IV or worse in women, particularly if present before the menopause – no other androgenization symptoms or signs. It is reasonable to carry out TT and DHEA-S, although some authorities suggest that these are more a reassurance to the physician than a clinical necessity!

- Severe hirsutism; female androgenetic alopecia – Ludwig III premenopausal or Hamilton grade V or more. These types are generally of greater significance endocrinologically if of rapid onset and continue to worsen. In the absence of other signs, DHEA-S should be done, as for group I – proceed to detailed ovarian and adrenal studies.

- Group 1 or 2 signs with disorder of menstruation. Any change in the normal cycle such as irregular or infrequent periods, and oligo- or amenorrhoea, or infertility, makes laboratory studies mandatory in all cases – proceed as for group 3 plus prolactin level. The latter may alter menstrual function without galactorrhoea. If LH and FSH are abnormal, then PCOD is the likely diagnosis. If amenorrhoea is total, serum oestradiol estimation is recommended.

  This group requires gynaecological assessment because of the risk of endometrial carcinoma.

- Signs of virilization. These include the development of group 1–3 signs, possibly with other skin signs such as acne, hidradenitis and prominent keratosis pilaris; also clitorimegaly, deepening of the voice and more masculine habitus. This suggests a

Table 7.2 Causes of hirsutism

Idiopathic (synonyms: cryptogenic or constitutional)

Ovarian
    Polycystic ovary disease
    Hyperthecosis
    Virilizing ovarian tumours

Adrenal
    Congenital adrenal hyperplasia
    Cushing's syndrome/disease
    Virilizing adrenal tumours

Iatrogenic

Hyperprolactinaemia

Hypothyroidism

severe central abnormality of androgen synthesis such as an androgen-secreting tumour. Investigate as for group 3 – all cases need to be assessed by an endocrinologist and a gynaecologist.

Table 7.2 shows the range of abnormalities that may be detected in patients presenting with cutaneous androgen-mediated signs such as hirsutism and androgenetic alopecia (mainly groups 3 and 4).

HAIR GROWTH METHODOLOGY

Length of the hair cycle: examination of hair roots

The length of the hair cycle can be studied by observation. This method relies on long periods of observation and accurate identification of individual hairs. It is more convenient to assess overall growth using hair length and daily linear growth (see below), in conjunction with assessment of hair root status. This gives information on the length of the growth cycle (anagen = total length/daily growth) and the percentage of growing roots.

Hair roots are examined by plucking hairs. The shafts should be grasped firmly and extracted briskly in the direction of their insertion. This ensures that the roots are not deformed. Surgical needle holders are used with the blades covered with fine rubber tubing or cellophane tape to ensure a firm grasp. Approximately 50 hairs are extracted in order to reduce sampling errors. The roots are examined under a low-power microscope (Fig. 7.1). The root morphology is stable and hairs can be kept for many weeks in dry packaging before analysis. Normal telogen counts are 13–15% on the vertex, but this figure will vary from site to site, with age, physiological androgen influences and many other factors. The appearance of the root is also important; shrivelled and atrophic roots are a feature of protein-calorie malnutrition.

HISTOLOGICAL TECHNIQUES

It is not always possible to get representative samples of hair by plucking, particularly when examining the balding scalp or assessing regrowth whilst the shafts are too short to grasp. In order to circumvent this problem, several investigators have devised histological techniques.

Kligman originally studied telogen effluvium by scalp histology, demonstrating increased telogen roots, in combination with a standardized combining technique and counting the shed hairs. These control data revealed that 90% of the normal population shed fewer than 75 hairs/day.

Headington made studies of hair roots using horizontal sections of scalp taken with 4–6 mm punch biopsies (Fig. 7.7). He defined the transverse appearance of the root in its different growth phases. Vellus hairs, which are defined as having a diameter less than 0.03 mm, are not seen below the entry of the sebaceous duct. Anagen hairs are recognized by the inner root sheath and absence of keratinocyte necrosis in the tricholemma. Catagen hairs have a thickening of the basement membrane in the lower external root sheath. Telogen follicles have a bulbous configuration and have no inner root sheath. With this technique, a 6 mm punch biopsy yields up to 30 follicular units or 80 terminal hairs. Once this technique has been mastered, considerable data can be gleaned regarding the total number and density of follicular units, follicular structures, their developmental stage and hair shaft diameters.

The estimation of root volume may be of more general use than the measurement of hair growth as the root volume and protein content are directly proportional, correlating well with reduction in body weight.

FOLLICLE KINETICS

Hair growth is the result of holocrine secretion by the hair follicle which occurs in bursts of activity. Therefore the direct measure of growth is by examination of the matrix kinetics. There are two methods of estimating kinetic activity – proliferative indices and metaphase arrest. The former is a count of the number of cells actually dividing at a given time; the latter is a count of the number of cells entering mitosis during a given period. The proliferative indices are the simplest and measure the proportion of cells at a particular phase within the cell cycle. The synthetic (S-phase) and mitotic (M-phase) are the most easily detected, being measured by the labelling index (S-phase) and the mitotic index (M-phase).

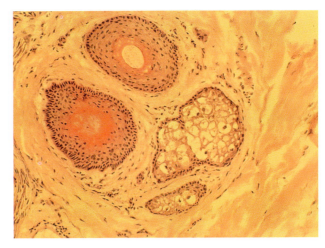

Fig. 7.7 Anagen and telogen follicles at the level of the sebaceous gland. Horizontal section; haematoxylin and eosin stain × 10.

Hair shaft length and diameter measurements

The hair shaft is measured using the parameters of length and diameter, and with these measurements the volume can be calculated from the formula $\pi r^2 l$, where r is the radius and l the length. The weight of hair is a comparable measure to volume but must be carefully standardized for shaving technique, washing and removal of epithelial debris. The easiest method to measure length is to bleach or shave the hair and measure the subsequent growth of undyed hair or stubble. Shaving does not have the advantage of removing telogen hairs. Plucking hairs is not a useful manoeuvre as it introduces a variable lag in growth until the shaft has grown through the skin, and animal experiments suggest that plucking may alter linear hair growth.

There are two widely used methods for measurement of linear growth – calibrated capillary tubes and macrophotography. Both of these methods are used after shaving, are repeatable and offer good correlation between observers. The capillary tube technique is easy and cheap, requiring only an accurately graduated tube (Fig. 7.8). Macrophotography requires apparatus to ensure that magnification and orientation are kept constant and that processing does not introduce any alterations in magnification. It does offer the advantage of clinical speed. The hairs are pressed flat against the skin with a microscopy slide to ensure that the entire length is visualized.

Hair clippings can be used to determine length or diameter and may be measured using a graduated eye-piece graticule mounted on a low-power microscope. Micrometers cannot be used as hair is too soft and will yield to low compression forces. The hairs should be mounted on a glass microscope slide using a drop of water or more firmly fixed with cellophane tape; Canada balsam or Depex – a high-viscosity plastic which sets as hard as glass on exposure to air – can also be used.

Compound measurements

The trichogram is a composite measurement of several growth parameters (Fig. 7.9). It was developed in order to formulate a more dynamic expression of growth. The term has been used by several authors to describe their different concepts.

Barman *et al.* described a less invasive means, involving multiple measurements which collate the number of hairs per unit area and shaft diameter, growth and root-cycle stage. A specifically designed microscope is used with 60 × magnification. This is placed on the skin surface which acts as the stage: two eye-pieces are used, one with a micrometer scale calibrated down to 0.25 mm and the other containing a reticulum defining an area of 4 mm². This area is then shaved and re-examined for length of growth after 5–10 days. Root status is measured, as before, by plucking. Using this technique, the investigators collected data on the normal pattern of growth in the newborn child, prepubertal children, adults, pregnant women, pubic hair and axillary hair. Stencils have been used to delineate the area to enable the method to be reproducible. This group also modified this trichogram by means of an intense washing and combing programme for 3 days, including the sample day, prior to plucking the hairs individually from a larger area of 35–45 mm².

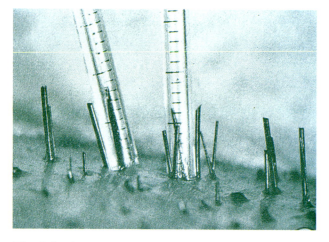

Fig. 7.8 Graduated capillary tube method for measuring linear hair growth.

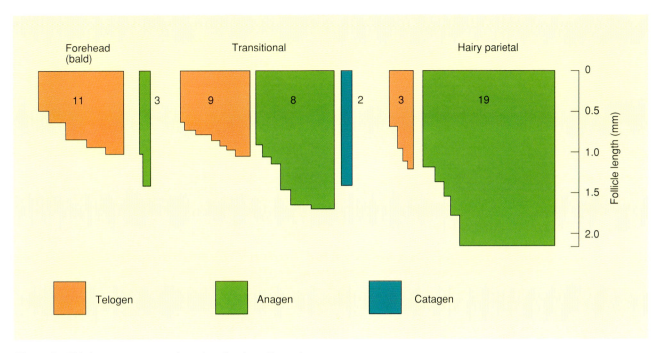

Fig. 7.9 Trichogram comparing density, length and growth phase of follicles at different sites on the scalp.

HAIR PLUCKABILITY

During studies of children suffering from protein-calorie malnutrition, it was noticed that the hair was not fully pigmented; it was thin, sparse, straight and easily plucked. Therefore, hair has been suggested as an easily obtained tissue source for assessment of protein-calorie malnutrition using anagen/telogen ratios, shaft diameter and bulb morphology.

A trichotillometer, a plucking device which comprises a springy dynamometer with a clamp to hold individual hairs and a scale graduated at 1.4 g intervals from 0 to 62 g, can be used to measure pluckability. The mean epilation force required to pluck 10 hairs has been assessed in normal and malnourished children and was found to correlate well with the serum albumin. The normal epilation force is >36 g, whereas in kwashiorkor it is <19 g. This measure correlates well with shaft diameter, which is also a good index of hair growth. Regional epilation forces have been measured for hair from the scalp eyebrows and cilia, and axillary and pubic hairs. However, this technique still needs to be rigorously evaluated on normal hair to determine variations with growth status (anagen or telogen) and with diameter.

Growth pattern analysis

In a human clinical setting it is useful to measure the changing pattern of hair growth. The patterns of androgen hair growth on the body (hirsutism) and on the scalp (androgenetic alopecia) have been formally defined, and grading systems formulated for the varying degrees of severity. These scores are easy to perform but are subject to considerable observer bias, as demonstrated in

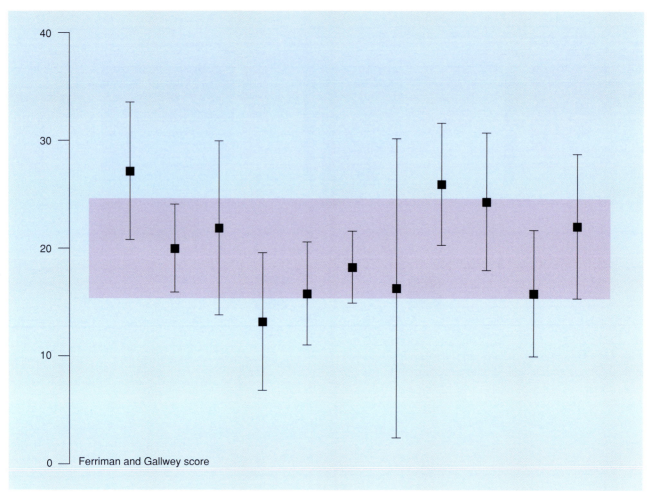

Fig. 7.10 This compares 11 studies which used the Ferriman and Gallwey scale to measure hirsutism; each is represented by mean ± standard deviation.

The wide variation in scores shows that no valid comparison can be made between these groups.

Fig. 7.10. This illustration compares the hirsutism score of 11 studies, all of which used the Ferriman and Gallwey system; the mean and standard deviation of each study are shown. It is reasonable to assume that the population of hirsute women presenting to any physician is similar and therefore no valid comparison can be made between these studies which have a wide scatter of values. This indicates that multicentre comparisons of therapies for androgenic alopecia or hirsutes cannot rely on subjective grading and must be supplemented with objective criteria.

FURTHER READING

Astore IP, Pecoraro V and Pecoraro EG. The normal trichogram of pubic hair. *British Journal of Dermatology* 1979; **101**:441.

Barman JM, Pecoraro V and Astore I. Method, technique and computations in the study of the trophic state of human scalp hair. *Journal of Investigative Dermatology*, 1964; **42**:421.

Barth JH. Investigation of hair, hair growth and the hair follicle. In: Rook AJ, Dawber RPR (eds) *Diseases of the hair and scalp*, 2nd edn. Blackwell, Oxford, 1991, pp. 588–606.

Caserio RJ. Diagnostic techniques for hair disorders. Part 1. Microscopic examination of the hair shaft. *Cutis* 1987; **40**:265.

Caserio RJ. Diagnostic techniques for hair disorders. Part II. Microscopic examination of hair bulbs, tips and casts. *Cutis* 1987; **40**:321.

Dupré and Bonafé JL. Pilar dystrophies studied by polarised light. *Annals of Dermatology and Venereology* 1978; **105**:921.

Ferriman D and Gallwey JD. Clinical assessment of body hair growth in women. *Journal of Clinical Endocrinology* 1961; **21**:1440.

Headington JT. Transverse microscopic anatomy of the human scalp: a basis for a morphometric approach to disorders of the hair follicle. *Archives of Dermatology* 1984; **120**:449.

Kligman AM. Pathologic dynamics of human hair loss. *Archives of Dermatology* 1961; **83**:175.

Ludwig E. Classification of the types of androgenic alopecia (common baldness) occurring in the female sex. *British Journal of Dermatology* 1977; **97**:247.

Saitoh M, Uzaka M and Sakamoto M. Human hair cycle. *Journal of Investigative Dermatology* 1970; **54**:6.

Schweizer J. Keratin expression in the human hair follicle. In: Van Neste D (ed) *Human Hair Growth and Alopecia Research*. Kluwe Academic, Dordrecht, 1989, pp. 11–27.

Simpson NB and Barth JH. Hair patterns: hirsutism and baldness. In: Rook AJ, Dawber RPR (eds) *Diseases of the Hair and Scalp*, Blackwell, Oxford, 1991, pp. 588–606.

Sperling LC and Heimer WL. Androgen biology as a basis for the diagnosis and treatment of androgenic disorders in women. I. *Journal of the American Academy of Dermatology* 1993; **28**:669–683.

Sperling LC and Heimer WL. Androgen biology as a basis for the diagnosis and treatment of androgenic disorders in women. II. *Journal of the American Academy of Dermatology* 1993; **28**:901–916.

Swift JA. The histology of keratin fibres. In Asquith RS (ed) *The Chemistry of Natural Protein Fibres*. Wiley, London, p.86.

Chapter 8

Investigation of nail disorders

David A. R. de Berker

CLINICAL EXAMINATION

Examination of an abnormal nail unit requires attention to detail. The digit needs to be assessed as part of a general examination and with reference to the other digits on the hands and feet. Scalp and mucosal surfaces require examination to exclude features of psoriasis and lichen planus respectively; these are common causes of chronic nail dystrophy. Further clues of an underlying dermatosis or collagen vascular disease may be present in the periungual soft tissues. The nail plate and underlying nail bed constitute a single unit for assessment of colour, as one can only be separated from the other by avulsion, which is seldom indicated. In the assessment of nail colour, there are several techniques that add to the potential amount of information gained. These need to be described in the general context of examination of nail colour.

Colour

Nail plate discoloration presents in three patterns:
- Total discoloration
- Partial discoloration with a proximal margin conforming to that of the lunula.
- Partial discoloration with a proximal margin conforming to that of the proximal nailfold.

Haem, melanin and leukonychia may present in a range of further patterns, not dealt with in detail here.

TOTAL DISCOLORATION

This may represent a persistent endogenous or exogenous cause, e.g. yellow nail syndrome.

PARTIAL DISCOLORATION CONFORMING WITH LUNULA

The lunula mimics the proximal margin of the nail matrix. Discoloration reflecting this structure indicates that the abnormality arose during nail generation, i.e. that there was an endogenous cause. The fact that there is now a proximal zone of normal nail indicates that the abnormality has passed and normal nail is now growing, e.g. true leukonychia.

PARTIAL DISCOLORATION CONFORMING WITH PROXIMAL NAILFOLD

This indicates that there has been an exogenous agent that has settled upon the nail some time before the assessment. Once time has elapsed, the zone of normal nail between the pigment and the proximal nailfold reflects the period of nail growth since exposure to the pigment. This can be used to date cessation of smoking with tabacco staining, or as a clue to treatment with potassium permanganate soaks (Fig. 8.1). With the latter, it is apparent that the thin cuticle extending over the proximal nail has less affinity for the stain than nail, allowing a thin rim of unstained nail during treatment.

Confirmation of exogenous pigment can sometimes be provided by scraping the nail. Whilst removal of the pigment confirms its exogenous origin, failure to do so does not necessarily disprove it.

Nail bed vasculature

The colour of blood in subungual vessels may lend a blue (cyanosed) or bright pink (carbon monoxide poisoning) colour to the nail. The nail bed may be coloured itself, as in minocycline staining of the proximal zone. The vascular component of any colour change can be assessed by two forms of pressure upon the nail unit:
- Vascular changes can be accentuated by having the patient press the pulp of the finger on a hard surface. This blocks the venous drainage of the nail through the vessels on the undersurface of the finger. The proximal two-thirds of the nail bed becomes more red. The distal component, corresponding to the onychodermal band, may become pale as pressure is transmitted to the firmly adherent overlying nail.
- Whilst the finger is kept in this position, blood can be prevented from entering the nail unit by pressing from above with a glass slide, resulting in pallor of the entire nail bed.

Transillumination

A small potent light source may allow transillumination of cystic structures of the nail unit. The only one of note is a mucoid pseudocyst, also called a myxoid cyst. Although this commonly occupies the proximal nailfold, this is not always the case. When within the proximal nailfold transillumination from a lateral site may be possible. When the cyst emerges from beneath the proximal nailfold, or is subungual, transillumination is technically impossible and of no diagnostic value.

Wood's light

In photo-onycholysis caused by tetracycline and demethylchlortetracycline, there may be a yellow glow to the nail when observed with Wood's light. This is normally combined with the clinical features of a scalloped distal onycholysis and brown nail bed margin. The condition spares the thumb and can be painful.

Wood's light may be positive in the examination of erythropoietic protoporphyria involving the nail unit.

INVESTIGATION OF THE NAIL PLATE

The nail plate is amenable to sampling without pain and provides the opportunity to examine pathological tissue in detail.

Microbiological specimens

PARONYCHIA

Acute paronychia is likely to yield *Staphylococcus aureus* or *Streptococcus pyogenes* when swabbed. It may be necessary to puncture the focus of pus formation to gain a specimen. This may also be needed to relieve pressure, which can cause pain and pressure necrosis of the matrix. The latter is a particular problem if infection primarily involves the proximal nailfold and there is a proximal subungual component. In this instance, a proximal hemiavulsion, or puncture of the nail overlying the matrix with a 4 mm punch biopsy (Fig. 8.2), under ring block may be necessary. Failure to relieve pressure can result in permanent nail dystrophy.

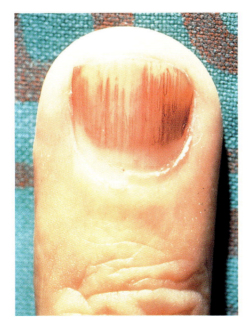

Fig. 8.1 Discoloration of nail plate with exogenous potassium permanganate: proximal margin conforms to the lunula.

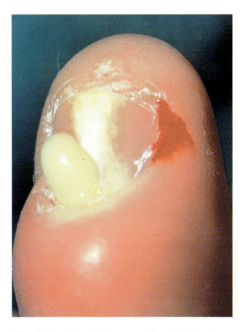

Fig. 8.2 Punch biopsy of nail plate in acute paronychia allowing decompression of the matrix.

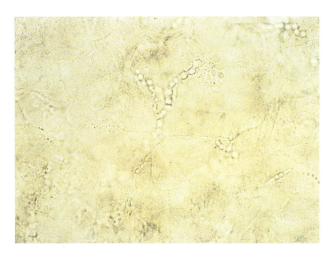

Fig. 8.3 Onychomycosis confirmed in clinic with potassium hydroxide preparation.

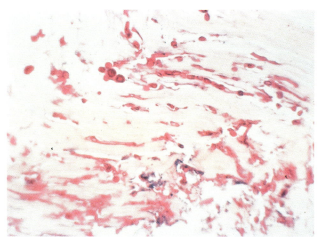

Fig. 8.4 Periodic acid–Schiff stain of nail plate section demonstrating fungus.

Chronic paronychia should be swabbed separately for aerobic and anaerobic bacteria as well as for *Candida*. There is often an element of chronic dermatosis which has been colonized and perpetuated by microbes, so that antimicrobial treatment alone may not be sufficient to resolve the condition.

PSEUDOMONAS

Green discoloration of the nail plate is usually associated with infection by *Pseudomonas aeruginosa*. This colonizes onycholysis which may be the primary disorder, which in turn is aggravated by infection. Swabs taken from an exposed nail bed, or the undersurface of a large nail clipping, may confirm the diagnosis. Suspension of the clippings in alcohol is said to demonstrate the soluble *Pseudomonas* pigment by changing the colour of the liquid. This distinguishes the green colour from that caused by serous exudate in psoriasis. This manoeuvre is difficult to perform successfully and it is preferable to have objective support for the diagnosis by positive microbiological culture.

FUNGAL INFECTION

The larger the specimen that is sent to the mycologist, the greater the chance of an accurate report. The specimen should include subungual debris as well as distal nail plate. The former often represents pathological hyperkeratosis and so provides a useful source of information. In superficial white onychomycosis, the friable white surface material should be sampled. Both forms of specimen can be examined in the clinic under the microscope in the same manner as skin scrapings. Material needs to be soaked in a medium that dissolves keratin and allows visualization of fungal hyphae (Fig. 8.3). There are several appropriate solvents:

- 10–30% aqueous potassium hydroxide.
- 12% potassium hydroxide in 40% dimethylsulphoxide.
- 50% Quink (Parker) ink in 50% potassium hydroxide.

Laboratory investigation includes the culture of crushed nail specimens. This is positive in only 55% of nails where fungi are seen on microscopy. Not all isolates are pathogens.

Nail plate histology

Histological examination of the nail plate may help in the diagnosis and understanding of several conditions. The most common instance is identification of fungi within the nail plate in nail dystrophies that are repeatedly negative for mycological examination and culture.

LIGHT MISCROSCOPY

Fungal nail histology

Hyphae can be seen within the nail plate when stained with haematoxylin and eosin, and with greater clarity when periodic acid–Schiff (Fig. 8.4) is used. Fluorescent lectin stains may further enhance the detection of fungi in biopsy material.

Locating the hyphae within the substance of the nail confirms that they are pathogenic. The nail specimen needs to be a clipping of at least 3 mm width. This can usually be obtained by large nail clippers from a long nail. Occasionally it may be necessary to obtain a surgical specimen under local anaesthetic. In this instance, a V-shaped nick can be taken from the nail tip or a 4 mm punch can be used at the same site. Any nail bed haemorrhage can be treated with electrocautery. There is no scarring.

Scabies

Both scabies mites and eggs can be found beneath the nail plate in Norwegian scabies. They may sometimes also be found there in less aggressive scabies. The reported specimens involve nail bed as well as nail, but this is not necessary. Haematoxylin and eosin staining of nail clippings may reveal parasites (Fig. 8.5). The presence of scabies at this site emphasizes how the scratching process is one of dissemination, with the fingernail as fomite.

Melanonychia

The clinical pattern of longitudinal melanonychia is usually sufficiently characteristic to allow exclusion of haem as the causal pigment. If there is doubt, there are three diagnostic options:

- The proximal margin of nail pigmentation can be marked with a groove made with a sharp file. The patient is then seen 2–3 months later. As long as the haemorrhage was not repeated, the pigment and scratch should move up the nail together, confirming the diagnosis of haematoma.
- A 4 mm punch biopsy of nail plate can be taken under ring block from the middle of the area of pigmentation. There will normally be a black residue on the nail bed.

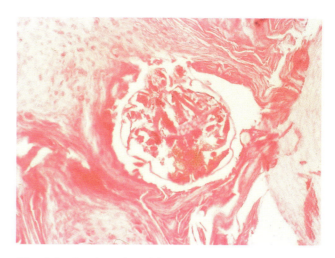

Fig. 8.5 Section of scabies mite within subungual debris in Norwegian scabies.

Any pigment of the nail undersurface will clear when it is cleaned in spirit. If there is any doubt, the nail can be examined histologically for melanin using a Masson Fontana stain. Absence of melanin excludes melanoma as the source of pigment, but its presence does not prove that the melanocytic lesion is malignant.

- Formal nail biopsy can be performed, to include nail matrix corresponding to the source of pigment.

Localization of the melanocytic lesion within the matrix

It may be that the clinician is in no doubt that the pigment is melanocytic in origin, and wishes to identify the location of the lesion within the matrix. This allows the surgeon to predict the degree of scarring likely with excision of the lesion. To comprehend this investigation it is necessary to understand that the proximal matrix produces superficial nail, and distal matrix, ventral nail. There is a proximal to distal gradient within the matrix that corresponds to a dorsal to ventral gradient in the free edge of the nail. When a nail clipping is taken from the free edge of a melanonychia, the site of the melanocytic lesion can be predicted if pigment is seen with a Masson Fontana stain (Fig. 8.6).

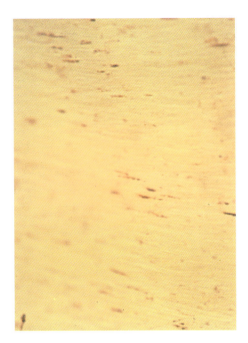

Fig. 8.6 Masson Fontana positive material present within nail plate.

Leukonychia

Leukonychia is seldom investigated histologically. When the nail plate is examined stained with haematoxylin and eosin, two features may be visible with the light microscope. There may be increased numbers of parakeratotic cells within the nail and there may be small splits within the laminated structure of this modified stratified epithelium. A small number of parakeratotic cells is seen in the normal nail, especially in the proximal, ventral region, where the residual nuclei are called Pertinax bodies. They are thought to be more visible when sections are examined using polarized light, but this is not always the case. Such nuclei may be more common in leukonychia.

Establishing the presence of small splits in the nail is also difficult. The action of the microtome on the nail plate can lead to artefactual splits, and any changes need to be interpreted with this in mind. Nail splits and increased nuclear remnants all contribute to altered refractive properties that might account for the whiteness seen in leukonychia.

IMMUNOFLUORESCENCE

Examination of whole nail unit specimens with immunofluorescent techniques can be a useful supplement to routine histology. The presence of immunoglobulin and complement has been confirmed at the appropriate epidermal sites in the nail unit in a range of immunobullous disorders. Nailfold biopsies in connective tissue may also be examined with immunofluorescence.

ELECTRON MICROSCOPY

The electron microscope is used mainly for research in nail examination. Transmission electron microscopy (TEM) can reveal changes in leukonychia and onychoschizia (lamellar splitting). In the former, there may be dense collections of intracellular material, interpreted as altered keratin. Onychoschizia can be induced experimentally by the repeated immersion and drying of nail plate specimens. Examination with TEM before and after this process reveals the separation of lamellae of nail correlating with the clinical appearance.

TEM, with uranyl sulphate staining, may also be used to provide a qualitative assessment of high sulphur protein in the nail. This is deficient in trichothiodystrophy, a syndrome where hair cuticle is weakened. In the scalp this manifests as alopecia. In the nail there may be koilonychia.

Elemental and constituent examination

INVESTIGATION OF DISEASE

Most nail constituent analysis is performed on normal nails in the context of systemic disease or poisoning. In children with cystic fibrosis, the chloride content of the nail can be estimated by X-ray diffraction and is found to be elevated by a factor of five above the level in controls. This has led to the proposal of screening for the disease, using nail by mail in regions where the sophistication of iontophoresis is not available.

Nail furosine (glycosylated keratin) can be estimated by high-performance liquid chromatography and has been shown to correlate well with fasting serum glucose. In diabetes mellitus, it provides a test comparable with glycosylated haemoglobin as a marker of long-term diabetic control. In a similar manner, Sudan IV-positive material in the nail can be assessed histologically and provides a guide to serum triglyceride levels.

INVESTIGATION OF EXOGENOUS MATERIALS

Industrial pollutants (cadmium, lead and zinc) have been measured in the hair and nails of children using atomic absorption spectrometry. This reveals the incorporation of these materials into nail and its potential as a guide to environmental pollution. Nail plate nickel has been measured by adsorption differential pulse voltammetry in a study of occupational exposure. It is advocated as a test to distinguish those with non-occupational nickel allergy from those where the allergy could be considered an industrial dermatosis. High levels of nail nickel suggest the latter. Nail drug analysis can be used for pharmaceutical investigation and as forensic evidence in instances of drug abuse.

PATCH TESTING

Patch testing should be considered in any nail dystrophy where there is periungual dermatitis, subungual hyperkeratosis, unexplained onycholysis or pain. The standard European battery should be combined with a cosmetic and medicament battery. Other batteries can be added as indicated by the person's history.

The pattern of digit involvement often gives a clue as to whether an allergic contact sensitivity is a possible cause (Fig. 8.7). Single-digit disease seldom represents contact dermatitis, unless there is a particular habit or occupation to explain the limited distribution. Generalized hand dermatitis frequently combines with nail ridging and discoloration secondary to chronic eczematous paronychia. Although this may be allergic in origin, it is a common appearance in endogenous and irritant eczema.

Allergy to quarternium 15, as a constituent of barrier cream, has been described as presenting primarily as a nail dystrophy. A more common source of reactions is nail cosmetics. Toluenesulphonamide formaldehyde is a constituent of most nail varnishes and some other cosmetics. It is a common cause of both local finger changes and eczema at other sites. The acrylates used in sculpted nails are potential sensitizers, although the original high-risk methyl acrylate is no longer used.

NAIL BIOPSY

Nail biopsy is amongst the most invasive forms of dermatological biopsy. The patient must be aware of the potential benefits of the manoeuvre and the exact details of the morbidity and long-term outcome. In a short text it is only possible to describe the more routine procedures. Patient preparation, anaesthetic (ring block with lignocaine or bupivacaine without adrenaline), tourniquet, postoperative analgesia and dressings should be arranged clearly and with care so that mishaps are avoided.

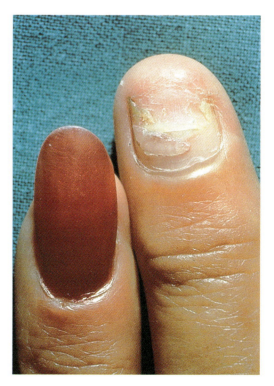

Fig. 8.7 Nail dystrophy secondary to nail cosmetic allergy.

Lateral longitudinal biopsy

This method of biopsy provides a representative section of the nail unit through all the main anatomical structures (Fig. 8.8). In doing so, it destroys part of the nail matrix and results in permanent narrowing of the nail. The lateral incision is placed within the sulcus of the lateral nailfold and extended through the proximal nailfold. The medial incision is placed parallel within 3 mm and brought around to meet the lateral incision at the distal and proximal extremes. This describes a thin ellipse which is then removed by gripping the distal end and dissecting the specimen away from the underlying bone, to which it is firmly attached. Particular care is needed at the proximal end, to avoid damage to the nail matrix, which may yield the most useful histological information.

The wound is closed with 3/0 monofilament suture. The direction of the suture is aimed at elevating the lateral nailfold to create a new sulcus into which the nail edge of the nail can be tucked.

Dressings need to be set out before completion of the biopsy so that there is no delay in their application. Otherwise, significant haemorrhage can occur between the removal of the tourniquet and dressing the wound. Materials should include an antimicrobial ointment, greasy tulle, absorbent

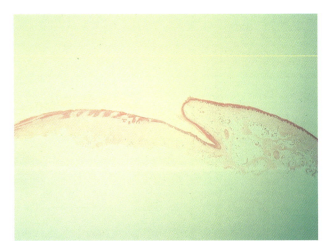

Fig. 8.8 Longitudinal nail unit biopsy through all structures.

padding and a bandage. Securing tape should not be circumferential as there is a risk of a progressive tourniquet effect upon the digit if there is postoperative swelling. Finger biopsies should be followed with a sling for the first 24h in most cases and the foot should be elevated for a toenail biopsy. Analgesia should be provided and if there are crevices or scope for contamination of the biopsy site, prophylactic antibiotics should also be given.

The wound needs review within 48–72h and sometimes earlier. Sutures are removed in 8–14 days. In the subsequent few weeks there is often scaling of the lateral nailfold, which should be treated with emollient to ensure a comfortable marriage between lateral nail and soft tissue.

Punch or transverse biopsy of the matrix

Punch biopsies (3 mm) of the matrix can usually be taken with minimal risk of subsequent nail dystrophy. This rule can be broken if the biopsy is taken very proximal within the matrix, or if the wound becomes infected. The biopsy may be taken through intact nail, or after visualization of the pathology following avulsion. The latter makes it easier to remove the small and fragile matrix specimen which is best handled with a skin hook. Closure of the matrix wound is desirable, but only possible if the nail is avulsed first. This should be done with a fine absorbable suture. If the opportunity to remove the suture subsequently arises, this may reduce the inflammation that degradation of the suture sometimes provokes.

Specialized techniques of matrix punch biopsy may be employed when attempting to determine the nature of a longitudinal melanonychia. This requires a sample to be taken from a point just proximal to the start of nail pigmentation.

Transverse nail biopsies may be taken from distal matrix with a reduction of nail thickness as the only lasting side-effect. The nail should be avulsed to provide access and the wound closed with fine absorbable sutures. This form of biopsy may be used in the diagnosis of a nail dystrophy, but the lateral longitudinal biopsy is usually superior in that it provides tissue from more sites within the nail unit.

IMAGING

X-ray

Plane and lateral X-ray of one or more digits in nail dystrophies may reveal characteristic changes (Figs 8.9 and 8.10; Table 8.1).

Ultrasound

Ultrasound is occasionally of use in the investigation of nail disorders. It has been used to estimate nail plate thickness with variable results. Myxoid cysts and glomus tumours may be detected with ultrasound, when high-resolution instruments are used in experienced hands.

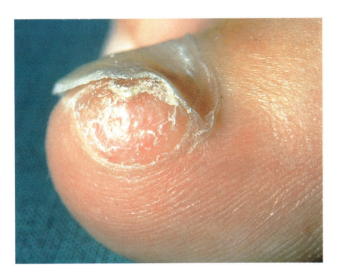

Fig. 8.9 Subungual exostosis.

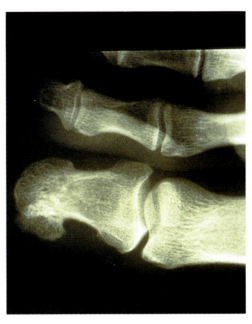

Fig. 8.10 X-ray appearance of subungual exostosis.

Table 8.1 X-ray findings in nail disease	
Disease	*X-ray changes*
Subungual exostosis	Cancellous bone tumour arising beneath nail distortion
Myxoid cyst	Osteoarthritis in adjacent distal interphalangeal joint
Glomus tumour	Bony erosion and star-shaped telangiectasis on arteriography
Psoriatic dystrophy	Bone resorption and destructive arthritis
Sclerodermatous changes	Acro-osteolysis
Clubbing	Acro-osteolysis or changes of hypertrophic pulmonary osteoarthropathy
Squamous cell carcinoma of the nail unit	Periosteal reaction of underlying phalanx
Systemic sclerosis	Soft-tissue calcification
Metastasis to the nail unit	Destruction of the distal phalanx

Magnetic resonance imaging (MRI)

MRI has been used to a limited extent in the diagnosis of site of lesions of the nail unit (Fig. 8.11). The majority of reports involve glomus tumours, where their subungual location, often involving the matrix, may warrant expensive radiological investigation before surgery. A recent survey of nail tumours examined by MRI described distinguishing features for glomus tumours, fibrokeratomas, myxoid cysts and subungual exostoses. The clinical value of this relatively expensive technique is not certain. The tumours examined in the survey are ones which are usually diagnosed on clinical grounds alone. However, it may be possible to delineate their extent preoperatively with MRI and so allow prediction of postoperative scarring.

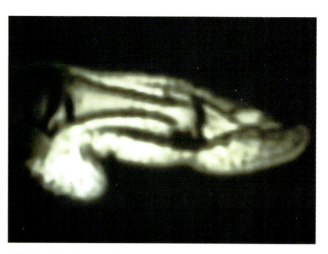

Fig. 8.11 Magnetic resonance image of subungual glomus tumour.

Photography

Photographic records are extremely helpful in the definition of nail disease and its change with time. This mainly reflects the difficulty of finding written terms that are adequate to convey the range and extent of clinical features present. A standard macro lens with extension tube and optional magnifying filter allow detail of individual nails and clustered fingers to be photographed with a single-lens reflex camera. A ring flash may fail to provide the flexibility of light source needed to highlight some details. A shadow-free image of a digit is produced by illuminating the field from the tip, shining proximally. This has to be done with a hand-held flash, which gives further options of oblique lighting and accentuating shadow when required.

A non-reflective background should be used, such as a fine-weave black or darkly coloured plain cloth. A slow (50 ASA) film provides greater definition than faster films.

Vascular imaging

Clinical assessment is the most basic and helpful form of vascular imaging needed in nail disease. More complex imaging is available, both with arteriography and methods of examining nailfold vessels.

NAILFOLD VESSELS

Collagen vascular diseases and Raynaud's phenomenon alter the capillary loops of the nailfolds and the structure of the cuticle. Detail of the capillary morphology can be examined using an ophthalomoscope or with a dissecting microscope if greater precision is required. In both instances, oil should be used to increase the lucency of the overlying epidermis. A photographic record can be kept using the appropriate attachment with the dissecting microscope, which allows progress of small vessel changes to be monitored.

The density of nailfold capillaries in systemic lupus erythematosus has been proposed as an indicator of pulmonary capillary loss. The loss of nailfold capillaries in systemic sclerosis has also been shown to correlate with systemic organ involvement. Typical changes in a range of diseases are described in Table 8.2.

Other methods of nail unit vascular imaging include laser Doppler and pulse oximetry. Laser Doppler flux metering has been used in sickle-cell disease where it is able to quantify reactive changes in vasomotor tone resulting in ischaemia. This has potential applications in the testing of

Table 8.2 Nailfold vessel changes in connective tissue diseases

Disease	Capillary density	Morphological changes
Scleroderma and CREST	Few visible vessels, with infarcted areas	Enlarged capillary loops
Systemic lupus erythematosus	Normal	Tortuous/corkscrew capillary loops
Mixed connective tissue disease and dermatomyositis	Few visible vessels	Enlarged, tortuous capillary loops. Features diminish with prolonged disease remission. Severity of changes in children may correlate with disease activity
Rheumatoid arthritis	Normal or few visible capillaries	Normal or irregular capillary loops
Behçets disease	Normal	Subungual flame haemorrhages or non-specific abnormalities
Hereditary haemorrhagic telangiectasia	Normal	Subungual telangiectases and haemorrhages, with giant capillaries in the proximal nailfold

CREST = Calcinosis, Raynaud's phenomenon, oesophageal dysfunction, sclerodactyly, telangiectasia.

therapeutic agents. Pulse oximetry has similar applications, as well as its more routine use in anaesthesiology and intensive care. This technique relies on the transparency of the nail. Coloured varnish and long nails cause problems in monitoring during general anaesthetic.

LONGITUDINAL GROWTH MEASUREMENT

The measurement of longitudinal growth in a nail may be used as a guide to the influence of systemic factors, such as age, sex, environmental temperature and diseases. Local nail disorders are only occasionally subject to this form of investigation. Yellow nail syndrome has been investigated in this fashion, to reveal that longitudinal growth rate is approximately halved in this condition. In cases where the diagnosis is in doubt, confirming this detail may be useful.

Most methods of measuring longitudinal growth involve making a fixed transverse groove on the nail at a defined point in the midline. This point may be defined with respect to the proximal nailfold or the lunula, if it is visible. Early studies involved placing bismuth amalgam in the groove and establishing its location with respect to underlying bony landmarks on X-rays. This is no longer acceptable, as it results in unwarranted irradiation.

In all methods, the groove needs to be sufficiently deep to remain visible throughout the growth of the nail. This is about 6 months in the finger and up to 18 months in the toe. Subsequent measurements are made of the distance of the line from the original reference point and total linear growth calculated.

FURTHER READING

Baran R and Dawber RPR (eds) *Nail Diseases and their Management*, 2nd edn. Blackwell Scientific Publications, Oxford, 1994.

Baran R and Kechijian P. Longitudinal melanonychia (melanonychia striata). Diagnosis and management. *Journal of the American Academy of Dermatology* 1989; **21**:1165–1175.

Chapman AL, Fegley B and Cho CT. X-ray microanalysis of chloride in nails from cystic fibrosis and control patients. *European Journal of Respiratory Diseases* 1985; **66**:218–223.

de Berker D, Dalziel K, Dawber R, Wojnarowska F. Pemphigus associated with nail dystrophy. *British Journal of Dermatology* 1993; **129**:461–464.

Hanno R, Mathes BM and Krull EA. Longitudinal biopsy in the evaluation of acquired nail dystrophies. *Journal of the American Academy of Dermatology* 1986; **14**:803–809.

Marren P, de Berker D and Powell S. Occupational contact dermatitis due to quarternium 15 presenting as nail dystrophy. *Contact Dermatitis* 1991; **25**:253.

Oimomi M. Maeda Y, Hata F et al. Glycosyation levels of nail proteins in diabetic patients with retinopathy and neuropathy. *Kobe Journal of Medical Science* 1985; **31**:183–188.

Robles MW, Boghal B, Morrell CA et al. The use of fluorescent lectins to identify fungi in clinical material from the skin. *British Journal of Dermatology* 1990; **123**:(suppl 37) 64.

Salamon O, Nikulin A, Grujic M and Plavsic B. Sudan IV positive material of the nail plate related to plasma triglycerides. *Dermatologica* 1988; **176**:52–54.

Tosti A. The nail apparatus in collagen disorders. *Seminars in Dermatology* 1991; **10**:71–76.

Wallis MS, Bowen WR and Guin JD. Pathogenesis of onychoschizia (lamellar dystrophy). *Journal of the American Academy of Dermatology* 1991; **24**:44–48.

Chapter 9

Prenatal diagnosis of heritable skin diseases

M. Giles S. Dunnill and Robin A. J. Eady

This chapter will deal with heritable skin diseases of sufficient severity to warrant prenatal diagnosis. These diseases are, in general, recessively inherited and rare, but will often present a heavy and long-term burden on the parents of affected children. Treatment is usually palliative. Rapid advances in the understanding of inherited disease at the molecular level will lead eventually to radically different treatments, but until these are widely available, prenatal diagnosis will have a significant part to play in disease prevention. Parents having had one affected child will often not wish to risk having any more affected children. Prenatal diagnosis can provide them with the opportunity of extending their family without this risk.

Knowledge of the normal morphology of fetal skin at different gestational ages, coupled with the development of fetal skin biopsy has enabled prenatal diagnostic testing for a number of different genodermatoses. This technique is now well-established. More recently, the explosion of research into the molecular genetics of heritable diseases and the powerful methods used in their analysis have provided the means to undertake rapid and accurate prenatal diagnosis using very small amounts of fetal DNA obtained early in pregnancy.

We will start with a discussion of the general principles of methods available for prenatal diagnosis illustrated by some examples. Specific diseases will then be dealt with. The rate of progress in this field is so fast that a detailed description of diseases currently amenable to prenatal diagnosis would quickly become out of date. The clinician faced with parents enquiring about prenatal diagnosis for a particular disease should liaise with local or regional genetics departments for up-to-date information.

METHODS

Fetal skin biopsy

Fetal skin biopsy has been in use since 1980 and is now performed in centres in the UK, USA, continental Europe and Japan. Worldwide experience in 1992 included over 450 cases. The main disadvantage is that it is not performed earlier in pregnancy than 15 weeks' gestation and is often done later. Mid-trimester termination of an affected fetus is thus inevitable when this approach is used. As more diseases become amenable to DNA-based diagnosis, first-trimester chorionic villus sampling should replace fetal skin biopsy. Notwithstanding, this technique still has an important role in prenatal diagnosis. It may be used for any disease in which the morphological or immunohistochemical abnormalities of fetal skin are well-established.

TECHNIQUE

The biopsy is taken transabdominally using high-resolution ultrasound scanning, under a local anaesthetic. Fine 20-gauge forceps are used to obtain small samples of skin (Fig. 9.1). Technically, the procedure is difficult to perform before 15 weeks' gestation. Gestational timing of the biopsy also depends on the disease at risk. Diseases such as junctional or recessive dystrophic

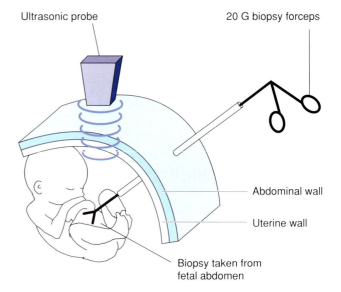

Fig. 9.1 Method of obtaining fetal skin biopsy. The biopsy forceps are introduced into the uterine cavity under ultrasound control. From Nicolini and Rodeck, with kind permission.

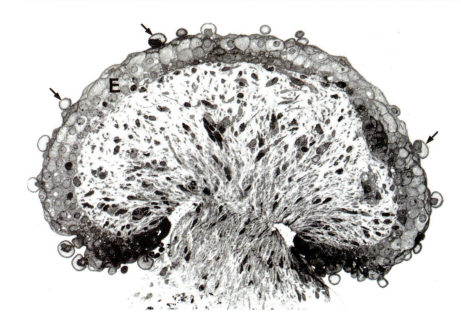

Fig. 9.2 Light microscopy of a skin biopsy taken from the buttock of a normal fetus at 16 weeks' gestation. The biopsy has rounded edges and a small stalk as an artefact of avulsion by the biopsy forceps. The epidermis (E) at this gestation consists of three cell layers and the periderm with characteristic blebs (arrows) × 120.

epidermolysis bullosa can be diagnosed on the basis of morphological and immunohistochemical changes which are evident at 15 weeks. Yet the abnormalities associated with harlequin ichthyosis may not be manifest until 22 weeks, and biopsy should not be performed before then. Thus the gestational age at which abnormalities can be detected reliably for a particular disease will also influence the timing of the biopsy.

The site of the biopsy is also important and will vary according to the disease at risk. Several sites should be sampled in all cases as relevant pathological changes should be demonstrated in at least two independent samples. This is particularly important for some forms of ichthyosis where there may be regional differences in expression of the disease. In tyrosinase-negative oculocutaneous albinism, the preferred biopsy site is the scalp (or eyebrow) to enable ultrastructural examination of melanosomes in hair bulb melanocytes. For other diseases, such as junctional epidermolysis bullosa, the site is not so critical and the biopsies are usually taken from the abdomen or thigh.

The risk of fetal loss following fetal skin biopsy depends on maternal age and skill of the operator. In experienced hands the overall loss rate is around 2%, which is 1% above the spontaneous loss rate at this gestation. Significant scarring resulting from fetal skin biopsy is rarely reported, and often the site of biopsy cannot even be seen.

SAMPLES

Where possible, several biopsies are taken. They are examined under a dissecting microscope immediately to ensure the sample is adequate and contains both epidermis and dermis. The samples are processed for electron microscopy and embedded into epoxy resin. Semithin sections can be cut, stained and viewed by light microscopy (Fig. 9.2). Ultrastructural changes can be detected by examination of ultrathin sections viewed by transmission electron microscopy. In junctional or recessive dystrophic epidermolysis bullosa, the trauma involved in taking the biopsy is usually sufficient to induce a split along the dermoepidermal junction. The level of the split can be shown on electron microscopy to be through the lamina lucida of the epidermal basement membrane in junctional epidermolysis bullosa, and beneath the lamina densa in recessive dystrophic epidermolysis bullosa (Fig.9.3). Morphological abnormalities of basement membrane zone structures can also be identified.

Fig. 9.3 Electron micrograph of fetal skin affected by dystrophic epidermolysis bullosa. Separation (star) between epidermis (E) and dermis (D) can be seen. The level of cleavage is just below the lamina densa (arrow) of the epidermal basement membrane. Bar = 5µm.

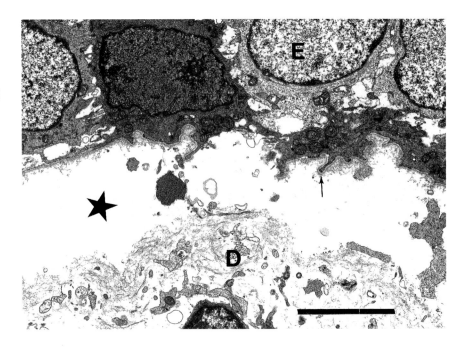

Samples may be snap-frozen for indirect immunofluorescence when specific informative antibody probes are available. For example, staining with antibodies against laminin 5 is reduced or absent along the dermoepidermal junction in samples from a fetus affected with lethal (Herlitz) junctional epidermolysis bullosa (Fig.9.4).

USAGE

The disadvantage of fetal skin biopsy, compared to chorionic villus sampling, is that of a mid-trimester termination for an affected fetus. By this stage the pregnancy will be clinically apparent to parents and others, and fetal movements will have been felt. Furthermore, the risk to the mother is greater for a termination at this later gestational age. One advantage of skin biopsy is that examination of a biopsy from the proband, although desirable, is not always necessary. It is unfortunately common for the first affected child to have died without either skin biopsy or DNA having been taken and stored. In these circumstances, it may be difficult to predict the expected findings on skin biopsy of an affected fetus, and impossible to apply the molecular approach (see below). Fetal skin biopsy has a good record of accuracy in junctional and recessive dystrophic epidermolysis bullosa. In a personal series (Eady and Rodeck, unpublished data) there have been no incorrect diagnoses. With the rarer genodermatoses, the figures are too small to draw any definite conclusions. Potential inaccuracies may arise from laboratory error or from attempting to make a diagnosis from a sample taken too early in pregnancy, before characteristic changes are evident.

Chorionic villus sampling

Biopsy of the chorion frondosum is now an established procedure and provides a source of fetal tissue from which DNA can be extracted directly. Cells can also be cultured for biochemical or cytogenetic testing. The ability to perform the biopsy at 10 weeks' gestation, combined with the speed and accuracy of polymerase chain reaction-based tests on DNA, means that the results can be available before the end of the first trimester. The number of conditions for which DNA-based diagnosis is available is likely to increase rapidly over the next few years.

Currently it is necessary to have DNA available from both parents and from a previously affected child before offering prenatal diagnosis to a couple at risk for any of the major genodermatoses. In cystic fibrosis, because common genetic mutations have now been defined for particular populations, it may be possible to perform prenatal diagnosis on fetal DNA without having examined DNA from a previously affected child. However, as yet there are no common mutations for the major genodermatoses so far considered for prenatal diagnosis, which means that DNA from the proband is still an essential prerequisite for DNA diagnosis of subsequent pregnancies. Testing is currently performed by research laboratories. For diseases such as the haemoglobinopathies, testing is routinely undertaken by clinical service laboratories, and in time this is likely to be the case for genodermatoses also.

TECHNIQUE

The biopsy is taken using local anaesthetic either transcervically or transabdominally under ultrasound control. Fine forceps or 20-gauge needle aspiration can be used. The choice of approach, and technique will depend on the lie of the placenta and preference of the operator. Biopsy before 9½ weeks may be associated with fetal limb defects and the procedure is usually carried out between 10 and 12 weeks. Also, there is an appreciable spontaneous loss rate before this gestation from karyotype abnormalities. Complications include bleeding, infection and maternal rhesus sensitization. Spontaneous fetal loss rate at this gestation is about 2–5% and loss after biopsy may be up to 1% greater than this.

SAMPLES

Fetal DNA sufficient for polymerase chain reaction can be extracted reliably from as little as 10 mg of chorionic villus (average sample size is about 50 mg). Chorionic villus cells can also be examined directly for cytogenetic abnormality or cultured for this purpose, but this may not be as accurate as amniotic fluid aspiration, especially if mosaicism is detected. Cultured cells may be used for biochemical and enzymatic assays. Tests for

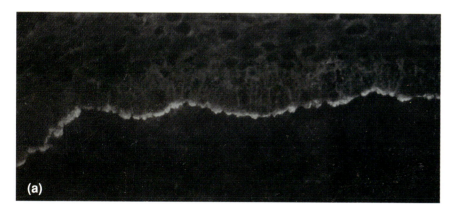

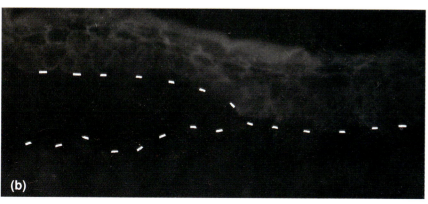

Fig. 9.4 Indirect immunofluorescence using the GB3 monoclonal antibody to laminin 5. (a) In skin from a normal fetal digit at 15 weeks' gestation, bright linear immunofluorescence in seen along the dermoepidermal junction. (b) In skin from the abdomen of a 16-week fetus affected by Herlitz junctional epidermolysis bullosa, GB3 staining is absent along the dermoepidermal junction (dashed line) where a cleavage has occurred. × 350.

light sensitivity and for deficiency in DNA repair can be performed in combination on cells obtained from chorionic villus samples in pregnancies at risk for xeroderma pigmentosum or Cockayne syndrome.

USAGE: DNA DIAGNOSIS

For a given disease, the elucidation of the molecular pathology generally progresses stepwise from finding the chromosomal locus of the gene responsible, through cloning and sequencing the gene, to defining mutations within that gene for individual families. The strategy for molecular prenatal diagnosis and diagnostic accuracy will vary depending on the current level of knowledge reached for a particular disease.

The locus for a disease gene is defined using **genetic linkage analysis**. This assigns the position of a disease gene to a region in a particular chromosome, defined by molecular polymorphic markers. The closer a marker lies to the disease gene, the less chance there is of a recombination between the marker and the gene during crossing-over in meiosis. When several markers are used, the site of the gene in question, in relation to the markers, can be accurately defined by testing for recombinations in families suffering from the disease. These polymorphic markers can then be used to form the basis of a molecular diagnostic test to detect affected and unaffected individuals using DNA samples. Note that in this situation it is not necessary to have cloned the disease gene, or to know anything about its function; the test relies simply on the knowledge of the gene locus. The phase of linkage (i.e. which marker allele segregates with the allele carrying the disease mutation) must be established in an individual family using DNA from father, mother and previously affected child prior to prenatal diagnosis. DNA from the fetus can then be assayed for the informative markers to establish which alleles it has inherited, and thus its disease status.

Once the disease gene has been cloned, polymorphisms, both within and tightly flanking the gene, can be identified and form the basis of more accurate markers. The marker alleles which segregate with the mutations in a nuclear family are identified and these can again be used to test the disease status of a fetus.

The most water-tight test of all can be performed if the mutation (or mutations) within the gene in both parents is identified. The molecular changes caused by mutations can often be used to design a rapid marker assay which can be used in combination with intragenic and flanking markers (Fig. 9.5).

PITFALLS IN DNA DIAGNOSIS

Although prenatal diagnosis using molecular markers tightly linked to the disease gene or based on the pathogenic mutation itself can provide extremely accurate results, it is important to be aware of potential sources of error, and of the limitations of these tests.

When flanking and intragenic markers are used without knowledge of the gene mutation there is a possibility of recombination between the marker and the mutation and so of misdiagnosis. When intragenic and flanking markers either side, and within 1 cM of the gene are used, the probability of error is less than 1%. In this situation we are also assuming that there is no possibility of locus heterogeneity (single disease phenotype which can be caused by mutations in different genes at different loci within the genome). One example of a disease which shows locus heterogeneity is bullous congenital ichthyosiform erythroderma. The same phenotype may be caused by mutations either in the keratin 1 gene on chromosome 12 or in the keratin 10 gene on chromosome 17. For an individual family it would be important to establish which is the causative gene before offering DNA-based prenatal diagnosis. Obviously, if markers for the wrong gene were used, the diagnosis would be incorrect.

The accuracy of the test also relies on the assumption that the paternity in the previously affected child and the fetus tested are the same. Non-paternity is usually apparent when using several diagnostic markers. Gonadal mosaicism in either parent, although a rare event, may also introduce a source of error. The rapidity of mole-

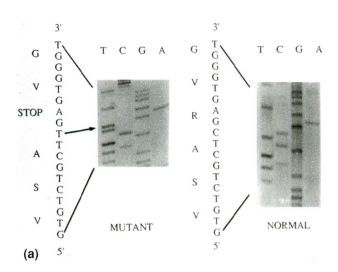

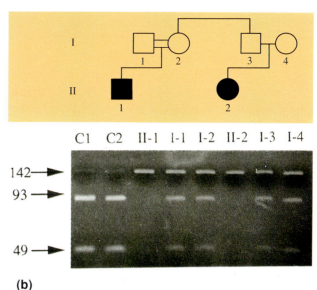

(a) MUTANT NORMAL

(b)

Fig. 9.5 An example of a mutation in the type VII collagen gene (COL7A1) causing severe recessive dystrophic epidermolysis bullosa. (a) The mutation, a homozygous cytosine (C) to thymine (T) transition, changes a codon for arginine (R) into a premature stop codon. This mutation abolishes a restriction enzyme site for the enzyme *Xho I*, present on the wild-type allele. (b) This restriction enzyme can then form the basis of a rapid test for the mutation using the polymerase chain reaction on small amounts of DNA. The results of the *Xho I* digests for the family carrying this mutation are shown. Lanes C1 and C2 are normal controls showing 93 bp and 49 bp fragments after digestion with *Xho I*. Only children (II-1, II-2) who have inherited both mutant alleles, as shown by the 142 bp band on the gel, are affected with the disease. Both sets of parents (I-1-4) are heterozygotes, showing all three bands. This test could be performed on DNA obtained from a chorionic villus sample from either mother to determine the disease status of the fetus. Open box = unaffected male; open circle = unaffected female; shaded box = affected male; shaded circle = affected female. Reproduced with kind permission from *Human Molecular Genetics*.

cular testing, which can be performed within 24–48 h, relies on use of the polymerase chain reaction. Sample contamination is a potent cause of error in any polymerase chain reaction and strict laboratory procedure, together with use of appropriate control samples, must be undertaken. Despite these misgivings, molecular methods have been used to provide rapid and accurate prenatal tests in cystic fibrosis, the haemoglobinopathies and many other inherited diseases. The same will be true of the genodermatoses.

Other methods

AMNIOCENTESIS

A sample of amniotic fluid can be taken at 16 weeks' gestation and will contain cells from fetal epidermis, gastrointestinal and genitourinary tracts and amnion. A proportion of the cells are viable and can be cultured for cytogenetic and biochemical analysis. DNA may also be extracted for polymerase chain reaction analysis. By far the most common indication for amniocentesis is maternal age. Sampling is routinely performed to detect karyotypic abnormalities. Fetal loss rate due to the procedure is between 0.5 and 1%.

Abnormal DNA repair may be tested by using amniotic fluid cells in pregnancies at risk for xeoderma pigmentosum. Metabolic disorders such as acute intermittent porphyria can be detected using enzymatic assays. Some cases of X-linked ectodermal dysplasia and incontinentia pigmenti may be associated with chromosomal abnormalities, and these could theoretically be detected on Giemsa or quinacrine band testing, although this has not been reported.

Various other abnormalities of amniotic fluid cells have been reported and may serve as adjuvant tests. It may be possible to detect abnormal keratinization in amniotic fluid cells in harlequin ichthyosis and in bullous congenital ichthyosiform erythroderma. Alpha-fetoprotein levels in extensive aplasia cutis congenita, from whatever cause, are elevated in amniotic fluid. Both these tests might give clues as to the diagnosis, but risk of false-negative results and non-specificity would rule out their use as the sole diagnostic test.

ULTRASOUND

High-resolution ultrasound is an important non-invasive screening test which is routinely used to determine fetal structural malformations. It can act as an adjuvant test to demonstrate polyhydramnios in pyloric atresia associated with some forms of epidermolysis bullosa, and in harlequin ichthyosis a 'snowstorm' appearance has been noted. These abnormalities may alert the obstetrician to the possibility of skin disease but would again not be sufficiently accurate to allow their employment as a definitive test.

MATERNAL BLOOD

Alpha-fetoprotein, a fetal product present in amniotic fluid, can be detected in the maternal circulation from the 10th week of pregnancy. Levels are evaluated in any condition in which fetal capillaries are abnormally exposed to amniotic fluid allowing increased transudation. Typically, this occurs in neural tube defects and assessment of maternal alpha-fetoprotein is used routinely as a screening test for these.

Intrauterine loss of cutaneous epithelia may also lead to increased levels, but this is neither sensitive nor specific. It has been possible to isolate fetal DNA using the polymerase chain reaction from a maternal blood sample as nucleated fetal red blood cells are present in minute amounts in the maternal circulation. These methods are not yet reliable, but could provide a non-invasive method of obtaining fetal DNA in the future.

SPECIFIC DISEASES

In this section we will attempt to discuss some of the conditions more commonly considered for prenatal diagnosis (Table 9.1). Many inherited diseases have some dermatological manifestations and coverage is by no means exhaustive. We have limited the discussion to diseases chiefly within the domain of dermatologists. The rapid progress resulting from research in molecular genetics is likely to change the possibilities for many diseases in the near future.

Epidermolysis bullosa

This group of diseases forms the bulk of referrals for prenatal diagnosis by fetal skin biopsy. Electron microscopy of fetal skin can be employed to identify the level of dermoepidermal separation and characteristic ultrastructural features in both dystrophic and junctional epidermolysis bullosa (Fig. 9.3). Furthermore, indirect immunofluorescence microscopy using antibodies against basement membrane zone antibodies can be used for prenatal diagnosis of these diseases (Fig. 9.4). Specifically, GB3 and 19-DEJ-1 show reduced or absent staining patterns in junctional epidermolysis bullosa. In recessive dystrophic epidermolysis bullosa, staining with antibodies against type VII collagen is reduced or absent.

Different genes at a variety of loci may cause the junctional epidermolysis bullosa phenotype and mutations have now been described in each of the three laminin 5 genes in junctional epidermolysis patients. Once individual mutations are defined it is possible to provide DNA-based diagnosis. Use of polymorphic markers without

Table 9.1 Prenatal diagnosis of the more common heritable skin diseases

Diagnosis	Inheritance	Principal method	Gestational age (weeks)	Skin/blood sample from proband
Junctional epidermolysis bullosa	AR	FSB CVS	15 onwards 10–12	Desirable Necessary
Recessive dystrophic epidermolysis bullosa	AR	FSB CVS	15 onwards 10–12	Desirable Necessary
Bullous congenital ichthyosiform erythroderma	AD	FSB (amniotic fluid*) CVS	19 onwards 10–12	Desirable Necessary
Lamellar ichthyosis†	AD	FSB‡	22 onwards	Desirable
Harlequin ichthyosis	AR	FSB (amniotic fluid*)	22 onwards	Desirable
Sjögren-Larsson syndrome	AR	FSB (Amniotic fluid enzyme assay)	22 onwards 16	Desirable Desirable
X-linked hypohydrotic ectodermal dysplasia	X-linked recessive	FSB	23	Desirable
Tyrosinase-negative oculocutaneous albinis	AR	FSB CVS	20 onwards 10–12	Desirable Necessary/ desirable
Xeroderma pigmentosum	AR	Amniotic fluid CVS	16 10–12	Desirable

• Amniotic fluid-derived cells, taken at 16 weeks' gestation, have been studied and shown to be abnormal, but not used as the sole diagnostic test.

† Lamellar ichthyosis is probably heterogeneous and includes alternative names such as non-bullous ichthyosiform erythroderma.

‡ Reported, but unreliable before 24 weeks' gestation.

FSB = fetal skin biopsy; CVS = chorionic villus sample; AR = autosomal recessive; AD = autosomal dominant.

knowledge of the gene mutation is not possible in junctional epidermolysis bullosa because of locus heterogeneity of the three laminin 5 genes, and the possibility that other genes may be implicated. Evidence so far suggests that all patients with recessive dystrophic epidermolysis bullosa have mutations within the type VII collagen gene (COL7A1). Intragenic and flanking markers for COL7A1, together with identified mutations, if these are available, can be used for DNA diagnosis.

Prenatal diagnosis by fetal skin biopsy has also been reported in epidermolysis bullosa simplex (Dowling–Meara). Now mutations in the keratin genes 5 and 14 have been defined, it would theoretically be possible to test for known mutations in fetal DNA obtained by chorionic villus biopsy.

The ichthyoses

These disorders are characterized by abnormalities of keratinization or terminal differentiation.

Diagnosis can be made by fetal skin biopsy, generally performed after 20 weeks' gestation, as this is when abnormalities become apparent. Bullous congenital ichthyosiform erythroderma can be done at 18 weeks and others, including harlequin ichthyosis, can usually be reliably diagnosed provided the biopsy is timed appropriately. Abnormalities in amniotic fluid cells may also be evident, but definite diagnosis still rests on skin biopsy. In lamellar ichthyosis (non-bullous congenital ichthyosiform erythroderma), there may be regional variation in expression of the disease with the possibility of a false-negative result.

Identification of mutations in the keratin genes K1 and K10 in patients with bullous congenital ichthyosiform erythroderma has allowed first-trimester prenatal diagnosis by direct gene sequencing. Recently, mutations in the transglutaminase gene have been reported in lamellar ichthyosis, creating the possibility for DNA-based prenatal diagnosis in this disease also.

In X-linked ichthyosis the steroid sulphate gene has been implicated. Enzymatic assays based on amniotic fluid cells have been used successfully in prenatal diagnosis. DNA-based tests using molecular probes for the steroid sulphatase gene are theoretically also possible. The Sjögren–Larsson syndrome, which has severe neurological features as well as skin manifestations, can be diagnosed on the basis of ultrastructural features present in fetal skin at 23 weeks' gestation. Another diagnostic test is based on assessing the activity of the fatty aldehyde dehydrogenase and fatty alcohol: NAD+ oxoreductase in cultured amniotic fluid cells, or chorionic villus cells.

Other disorders

A number of tests have been developed for tyrosinase-negative oculocutaneous albinism. Detection of stage III and IV melanosomes in hair bulb melanocytes can be enhanced by the dopa reaction test which may allow areas of skin to be sampled other than scalp. More recently, molecular analysis of the tyrosinase gene has enabled early prenatal diagnosis on chorionic villus samples. The biochemical and molecular defects of the tyrosinase-positive subtypes of oculocutaneous albinism are becoming clearer and prenatal diagnostic tests based on knowledge of the molecular genetics may soon be available.

X-linked hypohydrotic ectodermal dysplasia has been reportedly diagnosed on the basis of fetal skin biopsy, but numbers are few and regional variability in expression of this disorder may produce a source of error. Both X-linked hypohydrotic ectodermal dysplasia and incontinentia pigmenti have recently been mapped on the X chromosome (incontinentia pigmenti may have two loci) and molecular prenatal diagnosis has been achieved using linkage markers for anhydrotic ectodermal dysplasia.

In xeroderma pigmentosum, DNA repair assays can be performed on chorionic villus or amniotic fluid-derived cells to detect abnormalities. The various genes responsible for this disorder and other metabolic disorders such as the porphyrias are now becoming well-characterized, paving the way for DNA-based diagnosis.

COUNSELLING AND ETHICAL ISSUES

Parents and doctors should carefully discuss the appropriateness of prenatal diagnosis in each case. The probable severity of the disorder in an affected child and the possibility of new therapies which may be available in the future should be taken into consideration. The risks of the procedure should be balanced against the risk of having an affected child. The aims of prenatal diagnosis and how a couple would plan to act on a positive or negative diagnosis should be defined. The likely action on diagnosis of an affected fetus would be termination of pregnancy, and this should be discussed. Prenatal diagnosis for couples unwilling to undergo a termination is not usually appropriate, although it might be felt useful in order to plan a difficult delivery to minimize trauma to the baby, or psychologically to prepare the parents. Parents should be informed as to the nature of the proposed test and the possibility of a diagnostic error. Only after parents arc fully informed should the decision be made to proceed.

THE FUTURE: NEW DISEASES, EARLIER DIAGNOSIS AND SCREENING

In such a rapidly changing field new discoveries can quickly change the doctor's approach. Developments in treatment of genetic disease may render prenatal diagnosis for a particular disease less appropriate. Prenatal diagnosis at the DNA level may become available for diseases hitherto not considered as candidates, such as Darier's disease, epidermolysis bullosa simplex and even psoriasis. Ethical debate may temper the speed of change in such cases. New techniques may obviate the need for diagnosis *in utero*. Pre-implantation diagnosis using molecular analysis of DNA from a single cell derived from the eight-cell embryo is now possible, albeit in a research setting. This may become more widely available in the future.

For all the conditions discussed in this chapter, prenatal diagnosis would be considered in the context of a family which has already had at least one affected child. Detection of carriers of mutant genes is possible for some common hereditary diseases such as cystic fibrosis. It might then be feasible to screen couples and offer prenatal diagnosis to carriers before they have had any children. Yet, the rarity of most severe genodermatoses, together with the absence of common mutations would make screening couples for these diseases highly impractical for the foreseeable future.

FURTHER READING

Christiano AM and Uitto J. DNA-based prenatal diagnosis of heritable skin diseases. *Archives of Dermatology* 1993; **129**:1455–1459.

Cleaver JE, Volpe JPG, Charles WC and Thomas GH. Prenatal diagnosis of xeroderma pigmentosum and Cockayne syndrome. *Prenatal Diagnosis* 1994; **14**:921–928.

Eady RAJ. Genodermatoses. In: Brock DJH, Rodeck CH, Ferguson-Smith MA (eds) *Prenatal Diagnosis and Screening.* Churchill Livingstone, London, 1992, pp. 503–513.

Eady RAJ, Gunner DB, Tidman MJ, Nicolaides KH and Rodeck CH. Rapid processing of fetal skin for prenatal diagnosis by light and electron microscopy. *Journal of Clinical Pathology* 1984; **37**:633–638.

Eady RAJ, Holbrook KA, Blanchet-Bardon C and Anton-Lamprecht I. Chair's summary: prenatal diagnosis of skin disease. In: Burgdorf WHC, Katz SI (eds) *Dermatology: Progress and Perspective.* Parthenon, New York, 1992, pp. 1159–1165.

Elder GH. Molecular genetics of disorders of haem synthesis. *Journal of Clinical Pathology* 1993; **46**:977–981.

Hahnel R, Hahnel E, Wysocki SS, Wilkinson SP and Hockey A. Prenatal diagnosis of X-linked ichthyosis. *Clinica Chimica Acta* 1982; **120**:143–152.

Huber M, Rettler I, Bernasconi K *et al.* Mutations of keratinocyte transglutaminase in lamellar ichthyosis. *Science* 1995; **267**:525–528.

Kouseff BG, Matsaki R, Stenn KS, Hobbins JC, Mahoney MJ, Hashimoto K. Prenatal diagnosis of Sjögren–Larsson syndrome. *Journal of Pediatrics* 1982; **101**:998–1001.

Lane EB. Keratin diseases. *Current Opinion in Genetics and Development* 1994; **4**:412–418.

Lo YMD, Patel P, Wainscoat JS, Sampietro M, Gillmer MDG, Flemming KA. Prenatal sex determination by DNA amplification from maternal peripheral blood. *Lancet* 1989; **ii**:1363–1366.

MacLachlan NA. Amniocentesis. In: Brock DJH, Rodeck CH, Ferguson-Smith MA (eds) *Prenatal Diagnosis and Screening.* Churchill Livingstone, London, 1992, pp. 13–24.

Nicolini U and Rodeck CH. Fetal blood and tissue sampling. In: Brock DJH, Rodeck CH, Ferguson-Smith MA (eds) *Prenatal Diagnosis and Screening.* Churchill Livingstone, London, 1992, pp. 39–51.

Rizzo WB, Craft DA, Kelson TL *et al.* Prenatal diagnosis of Sjögren–Larsson syndrome using enzymatic methods. *Prenatal Diagnosis* 1994; **14**:577–581.

Rodeck CH. Prenatal diagnosis of epidermolysis bullosa. In: Priestly GC, Tidman MJ, Weiss JB, Eady RAJ (eds) *Epidermolysis Bullosa: A Comprehensive Review of Classification, Management and Laboratory Studies.* DEBRA, Crowthorne, Berkshire, 1990, pp. 10–12.

Rodeck CH, Eady RAJ and Gosden CM. Prenatal diagnosis of epidermolysis bullosa letalis. *Lancet* 1980; **i**:949–952.

Rothnagel JA, Longley MA, Holder RA, Kuster W and Roop DR. Prenatal diagnosis of epidermolytic hyperkeratosis by direct gene sequencing. *Journal of Investigative Dermatology* 1994; **102**:13–16.

Sassa S, Solish G, Levere RD and Kappas A. Studies in porphyria IV. Expression of the gene defect of acute intermittent porphyria in cultured skin fibroblasts and amniotic cells: prenatal diagnosis of the porphyria trait. *Journal of Experimental Medicine* 1975; **142**:722–731.

Shimizu H, Niizeki H, Suzumori K *et al.* Prenatal diagnosis of oculocutaneous albinism by analysis of the fetal tyrosinase gene. *Journal of Investigative Dermatology* 1994; **103**:104–106.

Silverman NS and Wapner RJ. Chorionic villus sampling. In: Brock DJH, Rodeck CH, Ferguson-Smith MA (eds) *Prenatal Diagnosis and Screening.* Churchill Livingstone, London, 1992, pp. 25–38.

Spritz RA. Molecular genetics of oculocutaneous albinism. *Seminars in Dermatology* 1993; **12**:167–172.

Zonana J, Schinizel A, Upadhyaya M, Thomas NST, Anton-Lamprecht and Harper PS. Prenatal diagnosis of X-linked hypohidrotic ectodermal dysplasia by linkage analysis. *American Journal of Medical Genetics* 1990; **35**:132–135.

Chapter 10

Molecular biology techniques in dermatology

Jane C. Sterling and Clive B. Archer

- **DNA and RNA**
- **General techniques**
  Electrophoresis
  Blotting techniques
- **Specific techniques**
  DNA cloning
  DNA sequencing
  Hybridization
  Polymerase chain reaction (PCR)
- **Genetic diseases**
- **Infections**
- **Cancer**
- **Inflammation**
- **The future**

No book on clinical investigation in medicine would be complete without acknowledgement of the potential role for the techniques of molecular biology in diagnosis and treatment. Some techniques currently used in the context of investigative dermatology will become the routine laboratory tests of the future.

DNA AND RNA

Molecular biology is a very broad term, encompassing the study of both DNA and RNA, which are the starting points for the production of proteins within cells, and also the application of techniques involving these molecules. In some ways the term is a misnomer, since the word molecular might readily be applied to other aspects of basic science research. In days when the attraction of large research grants is uppermost in the minds of those involved in medical research, the phrase 'using recently developed molecular biology techniques' perhaps helps to convey an image of research at the cutting edge. The whole subject began in the 1950s when the structure of DNA was described, but it was not until the 1970s that DNA and, later, RNA molecules could be manipulated in ways which allowed cutting, rejoining or copying of the strands, and the process of genetic engineering was born. In order to understand precisely how molecular biology can aid the diagnosis and treatment of skin disorders, it is essential first to have a clear idea of the techniques which can be applied and the basic science underlying them.

To revise one's medical school biochemistry, DNA is built up of four nucleotide bases, adenine, cytosine, guanine and thymine, which have the ability to attach together via a backbone of sugar and phosphate to form long strings and also to pair or **hybridize** via hydrogen bonds with one other nucleotide (Fig. 10.1). The long single strand is a fairly stable structure, but the point of pairing together with another strand is less strong. As a result, the two strands of DNA may, under appropriate conditions, separate and then possibly rejoin. In cells, the DNA is bunched together with proteins called **histones** to form

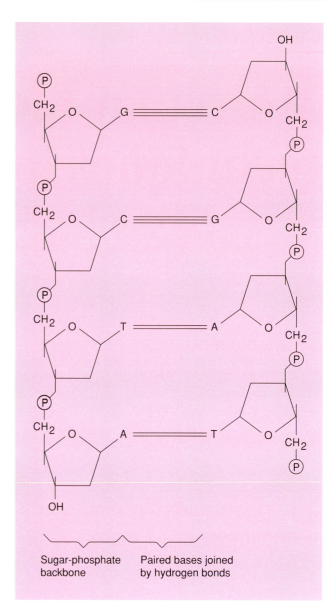

Fig. 10.1 Basic structure of double-stranded DNA. Bases (A = adenine; C = cytosine; G = guanidine; T = thymine) linked in pairs by hydrogen bonds and via a sugar–phosphate backbone.

the chromosomes. When cells divide, the chromosomes temporarily unravel during the formation of identical copies of the DNA (**replication**), a process that ensures that the genetic material of the DNA in the daughter cell is an exact replica of that in the parent cell. The production of protein

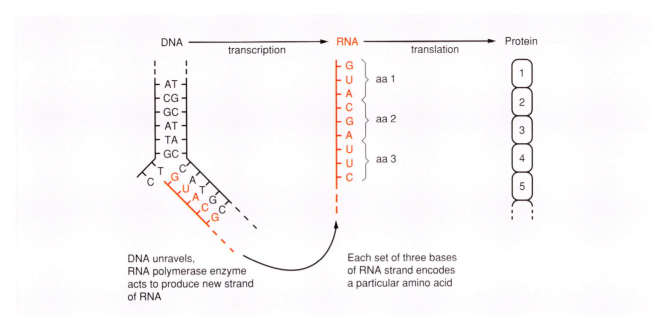

Fig. 10.2 Transcription and translation. Double-stranded DNA partially unwinds, allowing RNA polymerase to produce single-stranded RNA from the DNA template. Groups of three bases on the RNA strand code for a particular amino acid which join together to form a polypeptide or protein.

from DNA involves the intermediate step of messenger RNA (mRNA) production. The initiation of **transcription** (the formation of RNA from DNA) is a process which involves several elements and is only now being clarified. However, in simple terms, the DNA partly unravels, then RNA polymerase enzymes facilitate the development of a new string of nucleotides from one of the DNA strands (Fig. 10.2). One of the bases, thymine, is not found in RNA but its place is taken by uridine. Each group of three nucleotides in a strand of RNA is called a **codon** and can be translated into an amino acid. Some codons are **translated** as a start or stop at the beginning or end of a string of amino acids, thus defining an open reading frame or length of DNA which forms a **gene**. The process of translation requires a ribosome which can run along a strand of RNA, recognizing each codon in turn and pulling in the appropriate amino acid which corresponds to that codon. This process results in the formation of a string of amino acids joined together, i.e. a polypeptide or a protein.

Study and engineering of DNA and RNA from human tissue must begin with extraction of the DNA or RNA from the cells, but once isolated in solution, it can be modified in a variety of ways. The major ways in which DNA can be used for investigation or diagnosis are outlined here.

GENERAL TECHNIQUES

Electrophoresis

The method of subjecting macromolecules such as proteins, DNA and RNA to electrophoresis in slabs of gel (polyacrylamide or agarose) is widely used in biochemistry and molecular medicine. Electrophoresis can separate by charge, size or sometimes by both.

Electrophoresis of proteins is undertaken in the presence of a denaturing detergent, sodium dodecyl sulphate (SDS), and is generally carried out on gels of polyacrylamide in the forms of thin slabs held between two glass plates. After electrophoresis, the slabs are normally stained with

139

Coomassie brilliant blue, which stains the protein bands. The technique is usually referred to as 'SDS-PAGE' – SDS polyacrylamide gel electrophoresis.

This technique separates proteins by size rather than by charge. Proteins treated with SDS are denatured and bind to the SDS in amounts roughly proportional to the length of the polypeptide. Large proteins have a high negative charge and small proteins have a low negative charge. Since electrophoretic separation depends upon both size and charge, all proteins tend to move with a similar mobility in the presence of SDS. However, the use of a gel such as polyacrylamide allows small molecules to move more rapidly than larger ones. This graded sieving effect of the gel electrophoresis achieves separation by size. This type of separation is analogous to that achieved by subjecting DNA or RNA to an electrophoretic current in an agarose gel.

Blotting techniques

Analysis of the structure of DNA in a cell nucleus makes it possible to know which genes are present in a cell, whereas mRNA analysis reveals which proteins are being expressed at a given time, that is, which genes are 'switched on'.

In the 1970s, E.M. Southern described a method of transferring fragments of DNA to nitrocellulose sheets and analysed them by hybridization to pieces of DNA of known base sequence. These were referred to as Southern blots. Subsequently a similar technique was used for mRNA rather than DNA, referred to as Northern blotting. Western blotting is the term used for the transfer of protein from a gel to nitrocellulose or a comparable membrane.

For Northern blotting, total RNA is usually isolated from biopsy samples or cells in culture, taking care to avoid destruction of RNA by ribonucleases from various sources (e.g. microorganisms). The RNA is then subjected to electrophoretic separation within an agarose gel. At this stage, a range of types of RNA of different sizes are spread out in the gel but are not visible. To avoid diffusions once the electrophoresis

current is turned off, the bands are transferred to a sheet of nitrocellulose membrane by 'blotting'. With gentle pressure, the bands of RNA are transferred or 'printed' on to nitrocellulose as buffer flows through the gel, drawn by very slow suction. RNA (and DNA) stick very tightly to nitrocellulose and the gel pattern can either be stored or used in hybridization experiments (see later).

SPECIFIC TECHNIQUES

DNA cloning

The process of DNA cloning has been central to the development of molecular biology. It depends on two main reactions which in turn depend on two types of enzymes: first, enzymes which can cut DNA strands at particular points, **restriction endonucleases**, and second, enzymes which can stick the ends of DNA together, **ligases**. Many bacteria are able to produce restriction enzymes and these are named according to the bacterial origin. Thus, for instance, the enzyme Eco RI was purified from *Escherichia coli* RY13, Bam HI from *Bacillus amyloliquefaciens* H and Sma 1 from *Serratia marcescens*. There are very many more such enzymes, each of which recognizes a specific sequence of bases within a DNA strand which it is able to cut. Bam HI will cut the double DNA strand wherever the sequence --GGATCC-- is found, leaving a staggered or sticky end, whilst Sma I cuts in the sequence --CCCGGG-- to leave a blunt end (Fig 10.3).

Once a long strand of DNA has been cleaved into fragments of various lengths, these fragments can be separated one from the other on the basis of size by electrophoresis through a gel made of agarose, since smaller pieces are able to migrate more quickly through the gel than longer lengths (Fig. 10.4). The DNA can then be extracted from the agarose and inserted via ligation into a **cloning vector**. Cloning vectors can be taken up by fast-growing organisms such as bacteria or yeast in which they will replicate along with the host cell. Thus, multiple copies of the vector can then be produced via the multiplication of the

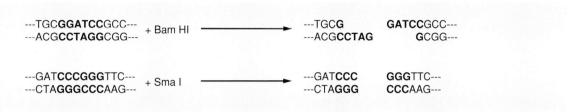

Fig. 10.3 Restriction enzyme digestion. Each restriction enzyme recognizes a specific series of bases, as shown in **bold** type. The action of the enzyme is to cut or cleave the double strand of DNA at a point in the series of nucleotides, leaving sticky ends (as with Bam HI) or blunt ends (as with Sma I).

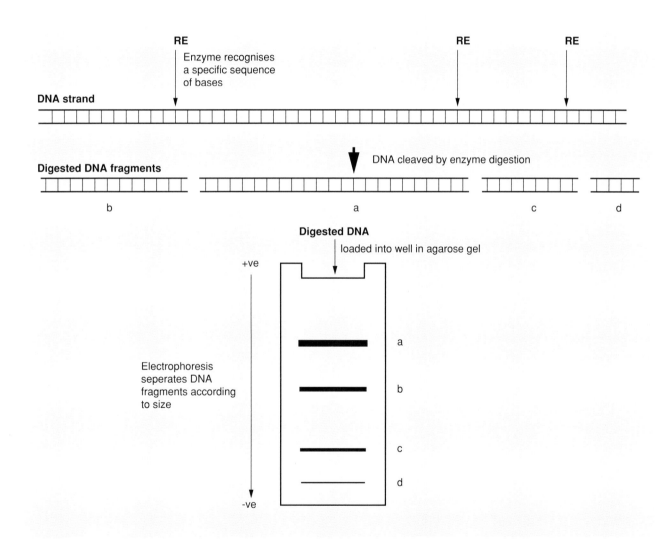

Fig. 10.4 Agarose gel electrophoresis of DNA cleaved by restriction enzymes. Long lengths of DNA are incubated with restriction endonuclease (RE) to cut the DNA at sites of specific sequence. The resulting mixture of smaller fragments is separated into its individual components by electrophoresis through an agarose gel. Smaller fragments of DNA migrate faster.

host cell. Cloning vectors are commonly **plasmids**, small circular DNA molecules which occur naturally in bacteria and are the means by which bacteria acquire antibiotic resistance. Such plasmids are now usually modified to make cloning easier by the insertion of specific short sequences of DNA which consist of a run of restriction enzyme cutting sites into which foreign DNA can be ligated. **Cosmids** (much larger constructs of plasmid-like DNA packaged within a bacteriophage or phage) and some DNA viruses can be used as cloning vectors and single-stranded DNA can be replicated via the use of a phage.

Cloning is the method most frequently used in the genetic engineering of proteins. For expression of a gene to produce its protein, the gene must be under the control of a **promoter** which will drive the RNA polymerase reaction. The addition of such a promoter sequence into a cloning vector just upstream of a cloning site where foreign DNA can be inserted leads to the formation of an **expression vector**. Promoters used in such systems are often inducible, that is, they may be turned on or off by physical conditions such as temperature or by chemical conditions such as the addition of specific molecules.

The proteins produced in this way can be used directly in therapy, for instance insulin and interferons, but may be used to produce an immunological reaction which will confer immunity. For instance, the immunogens used recently to produce immunity to hepatitis A or B are all products of genetic engineering. In the specific terms of the diagnosis of skin disorders or other diseases however, cloned proteins are now a very frequent source of immunogen used for the production of antibodies needed for diagnostic tests. The use of cloned proteins as immunogens allows specificity of the antibody response. If the genetic sequence of the gene is already known, an alternative means of producing a specific immunogen is via the mechanical synthesis of peptides. Peptide synthesis may circumvent the need for cloning in some circumstances; not only in the production of antibodies but also in the verification of which precise area of a protein is recognized by an antibody.

DNA sequencing

Knowledge of the precise order of bases within a gene or even an entire organism adds a huge benefit in terms of understanding the nature of the protein produced from a gene, how the expression of such a protein may be controlled and how organisms may be related to each other. The vast international Human Genome Project which plans to sequence the entire human genome is evidence of the importance of this technique.

The most commonly used method of sequencing is based on that developed by Sanger in 1977. It involves the use of a '**primer**', a short length of chemically synthesized single-stranded DNA of known base order which is homologous to the sequence at one end of the strand of interest. This area of homology to the primer is often chosen to be within the vector into which the strand of DNA has been cloned. The DNA to be sequenced must first be made single-stranded by heating or by treatment with alkali and then the primer is allowed to **anneal** or stick via hydrogen bonding to the area of its complementary bases. With the addition of a mixture of all the bases and the enzyme DNA polymerase, a chain extension reaction can occur which results in the production of a new strand of DNA complementary to the original.

In order to be able to ascertain the order in which bases are added, the reaction is modified in two ways. First, the reaction mixture is divided into four portions, each of which has a slightly different composition of nucleotides which includes a chain-terminating version of one of the bases, the dideoxy-base. Thus, the presence of dideoxy-adenosine triphosphate, ddATP, in a mixture which already contains all the four bases in the deoxy form, results in the variable incorporation of the dideoxy version of the base at intervals in the polymerase reaction (Fig. 10.5). The reaction cannot proceed past the dideoxy base and therefore terminates at that site. Because dATP is also present as well as ddATP, several different reaction products will be formed, each of which will terminate at a ddATP. The second modification allows visualization of the reaction

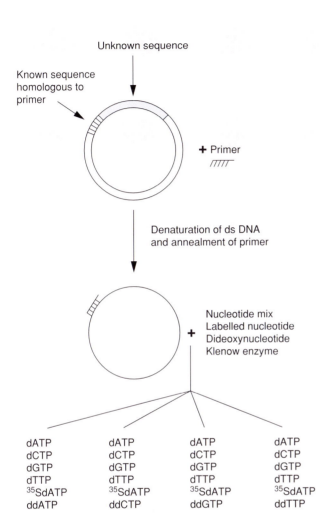

Extension reaction
in presence of:
Mixture of oligonucleotides
labelled oligonucleotide
one dideoxynucleotide
polymerase enzyme

Mixture of extension reaction products of differing lengths
according to site of incorporating the dideoxynucleotide, with
incorporated labelled nucleotide.

Priming oligonucleotide

Radiolebelled deoxynucleotide

Chain terminating dideoxynucleotide

Reaction products separated according
to size in a polyacrylamide gel.
Each track contains the results of
termination by one of the dideoxynucleotides

T   C   G   A

Reading from top to bottom i.e.
shortest to longest extension product.
the sequence is:

TCCTGAAACTGCACCGTCGGATGC

Fig. 10.5 The sequencing reaction. For each length of DNA and its specific primer, four reactions are performed with the four different types of chain-terminating dideoxynucleotides. ds = Double-stranded.

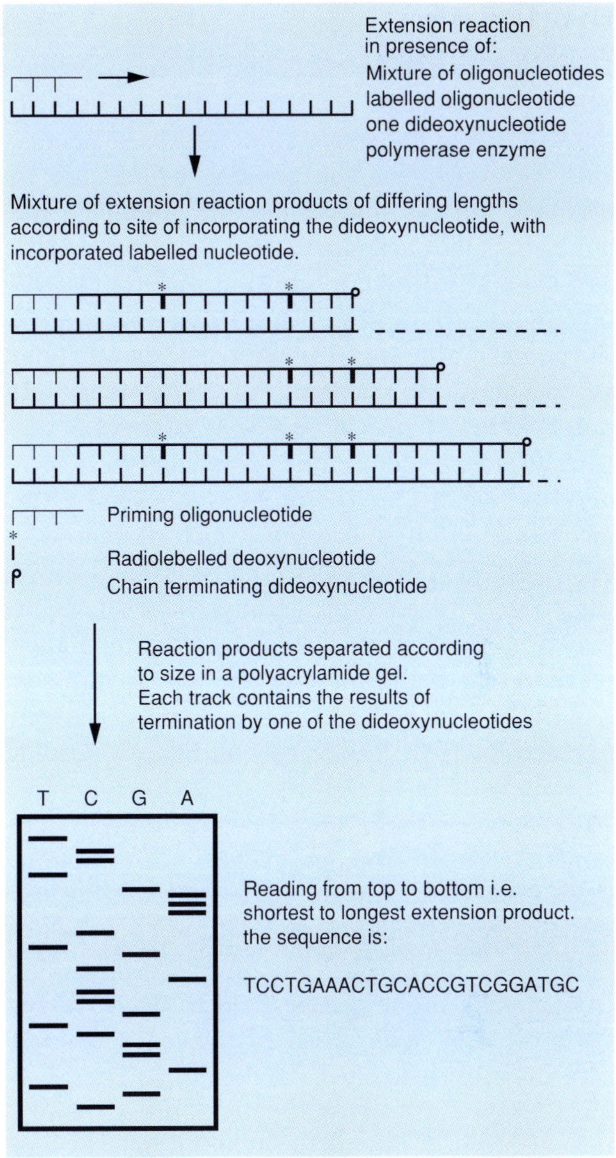

Fig. 10.6 Reading a sequence. Each of the four different reaction mixtures will contain extension products which terminate with the particular dideoxynucleotide. The mixture of different-sized lengths of DNA are separated according to size (i.e. length) by electrophoresis.

products. This is achieved by the incorporation of a radiolabelled (usually ^{35}S) version of one of the bases into the mixture. If ^{35}S dATP is used, this will be added to the extension product instead of the unlabelled dATP at some points.

The four different reaction mixtures are allowed to proceed with the extension reaction for just a few minutes before this is stopped and the mixture of reaction products then separated by electrophoresis in a long polyacrylamide gel. The gel is then 'read' to ascertain the order of bases (Fig. 10.6).

Hybridization

The technique of hybridization is central to the detection of specific portions of DNA or RNA. It relies on the innate tendency of lengths of DNA or RNA to anneal via the bonding of adenine to thymine and cytosine to guanine producing the double strands of a ladder formation. The physical and chemical conditions around the strands will favour either annealing or **melting** (separation of the strands) and so can be altered sequentially to allow a series of reactions. Diagnostic hybridization involves the use of a probe of known DNA or RNA to detect identical or complementary DNA or RNA (Fig. 10.7). The probe is labelled by the incorporation of a base to which is bound a detectable molecule. This could be a radioisotope (detectable by autoradiography) or a molecule which can be detected directly by a colour change reaction (e.g. biotin) or indirectly via an antibody (e.g. digoxigenin). The labelled probe is allowed to react slowly with the target nucleic acid until it anneals with it. In the case of DNA probe and DNA target, both must be denatured, i.e. rendered single-stranded, before the reaction. RNA, however, is already single-stranded, but the reaction conditions are slightly altered to allow annealing.

A labelled probe can be used to detect target DNA or RNA which has first, been separated according to size in a gel and then transferred to a nitrocellulose or nylon filter (Southern blot); second, dotted on to a filter (filter *in situ* hybridization, FISH); or third, left *in situ* in cells in culture or in tissue sections (*in situ* hybridization; Fig. 10.8).

Polymerase chain reaction (PCR)

PCR is a very powerful technique in which a small amount of DNA can be multiplied into a very much larger quantity. PCR is similar in many respects to the basic reaction which is used in sequencing in that a chain extension aided by the polymerase enzyme is of crucial importance.

The ability to perform PCR depends on two essential elements: the knowledge of the sequence of the DNA at either end of the length

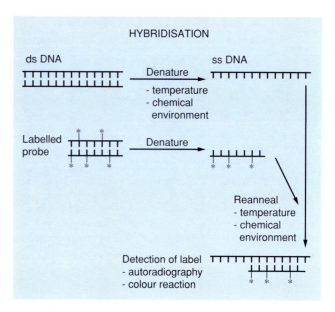

Fig. 10.7 Hybridization. The single-stranded labelled probe can hybridize to RNA or single-stranded DNA and the label indicates the site of the nucleic acid to which it has annealed.

which is to be amplified and the polymerase enzyme necessary to drive the reaction. Two **primers**, short lengths of single-stranded DNA (oligonucleotides), complementary to parts at each end but on different strands of the DNA to be amplified, must be synthesized.

DNA which contains or which may contain the sequence of interest is mixed with two olignucleotide primers, the polymerase enzyme and appropriate chemicals to buffer the reaction. By a repeated series of three temperature alterations, thermal **cycling**, the DNA will melt, the oligonucleotides will then have the opportunity to anneal to the complementary site on the DNA and the polymerase reaction can proceed (Fig. 10.9). These three steps are repeated many times, perhaps 20–40 times, thus amplifying what may have started off as only a relatively few copies of DNA into many thousands of copies which can of course be much more readily detected and subsequently analysed. If only one single copy of the strand of DNA in question was present at the start of the reaction, after 10 cycles this would have been amplified to 1024 copies, and after 20 cycles,

1 048 576 copies would have been produced.

The power of this technique does bring some problems. First, it is very easy for contamination to occur within a laboratory in which instruments are used for a variety of purposes and in which several molecular processes may be in use at any one time. This can lead to false-positive reactions. Second, there may be non-specific binding of the primers to unintended sites. This will lead to the amplification of the wrong product. Nested PCR involves standard PCR followed by a second reaction using a different pair of primers which bind inside the original pair. This modification increases the sensitivity of the amplification, since for the second product to be made, the first product must be the correct one. The second reaction would not be able to occur if the primers had bound at a site other than the expected site and had produced strands of DNA which did not correspond to the sequence sought.

RNA can also be detected by PCR, but only with an additional initial step in which the RNA is copied into a DNA strand by the enzyme **reverse transcriptase**. The DNA produced by this reaction can then be subjected to amplification by PCR. This adaptation of the techniques is known as reverse transcription PCR (RT PCR).

GENETIC DISEASES

Within the human genome, a single alteration in a nucleotide base pair within a gene encoding a protein can produce derangements of function which lead to disease. Such a mutation in the DNA sequence can arise spontaneously, but may then be passed from parent to child. Diseases which run in families are likely to be caused by a genetic abnormality and such families form the starting point for the investigation of the responsible gene.

Such a study begins with **linkage analysis**, which depends on the fact that cross-over of chromosomal DNA between alleles can occur during meiotic cell division. Regions in close proximity on a chromosome are unlikely to be separated by cross-over, whilst a large distance between two regions will favour the chances of separation. DNA, usually obtained from lymphocytes, is collected from several affected and unaffected family members. The DNA is divided and each aliquot digested with a different restriction enzyme. When the DNA fragments are separated on an agarose gel, the pattern produced can be compared between individuals (Fig. 10.10). With luck, a particular enzyme will produce a fragment of consistently longer or shorter length in the affected than in the unaffected individuals, i.e. a **restriction fragment length polymorphism** or RFLP. This step identifies an area of the genome of several thousand base pairs near which the gene lies. The next stage is to identify the chromosome on which the gene resides and then the gene itself.

Once a gene is potentially identified, the possible mutation has to be ascertained by extensive sequencing of the **candidate gene** in both affected and unaffected individuals. There may be several different ways in which the gene may be mutated to produce a functional abnormality of the protein it encodes. As a further check, transgenic mice may be produced in which the mutated gene is cloned into the germ line of mice and the effect on the animal observed.

The rare autosomal dominant disease epidermolysis bullosa simplex of the Dowling–Meara type, in which blisters form on the skin after mild friction, has been defined in terms of the genetic mutation. In family studies, epidermolysis bullosa simplex was initially shown to be linked to the chromosomes carrying the keratin genes, namely chromosomes 17 and 12. Coincidentally, a mutated keratin type 14 was used to make a transgenic mouse, which showed changes of skin fragility and blistering with histological features similar to those found in the human disease. Finally, a series of patients was subsequently examined and found to have mutations in the keratin 5 or keratin 14 genes, which encode the two major keratins found in the cells of the basal layer of the epidermis. The slightly abnormal keratins formed by the mutated genes are not able to build a strong filament network within the basal cells, which then tear apart under pressure or shearing force, leading to blistering.

INFECTIONS

As discussed in Chapter 6, molecular techniques can be very usefully applied to the detection of foreign DNA or RNA from pathogens in tissue or fluid and are now often used in the identification of infectious agents. The use of hybridization or PCR may be much more rapid than the more traditional methods of culture of organisms and may even allow both diagnosis and typing at the same time. For instance, the presence of herpesvirus can be shown very quickly by electron microscopy of blister fluid, but since all viruses of the herpes group look very similar, it would not be possible to distinguish between herpes simplex types 1 and 2, or varicella-zoster virus. However, PCR of blister fluid using type-specific oligonucleotide primers would take 3–4 h and would allow distinction between the possibilities. An alternative approach to rapid diagnosis of different herpes simplex types is the application of immunocytochemistry using antibodies prepared against cloned viral proteins which are specific for the different types.

In some instances, variations in pathogenic organisms are detectable only by molecular techniques and not by immunology. The human papillomavirus (HPV) family consists of over 70 different types, although in practice the common skin and mucosal warts are caused by only a small number of these different types. In order to identify precisely which HPV type is present within a lesion, it would be necessary either to extract the DNA for analysis by hybridization or PCR or to perform *in situ* hybridization on tissue sections (Fig. 10.8). This sort of investigation might be considered when a child presents with genital warts and when sexual abuse is thought to be a possibility. Typing of the HPV in the child's lesions would show if the warts were caused by the HPV types, which also cause genital warts in adults and if so, if they contained exactly the same type present in any adult whom the child has close contact. The finding of such a correlation would not be proof of abuse since genital-associated HPVs can be transmitted non-sexually, and would only act as one piece of evidence.

DNA detection by PCR and then hybridization to check specificity of the reaction is also very useful diagnostically in situations where the

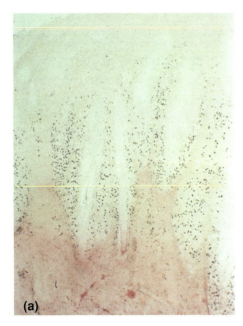

(a)

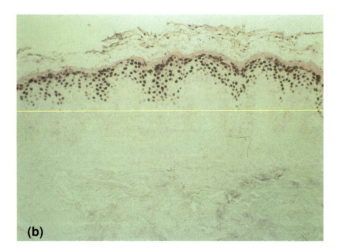

(b)

Fig. 10.8 *In situ* hybridization of viral DNA within cutaneous warts. The tissue sections have been allowed to react with a probe labelled with digoxigenin. The digoxigenin is then localized by a labelled monoclonal antibody and followed by a colour change reaction. (a) Hyperkeratotic wart following hybridization with human papillomavirus (HPV) type 2 probe. (b) Plane wart following hybridization with HPV type 3 probe.

infecting organism grows poorly in culture. For example, mycobacteria can be notoriously difficult to identify, requiring repeated sample collection and sensitive culture conditions. PCR of either sputum or blood can give a much quicker positive answer, although the presence of DNA of *Mycobacterium tuberculosis* in the sputum may not distinguish between active tuberculosis and tuberculosis which is under treatment but no longer infectious. Cutaneous infection with *M. marinum* cannot yet be diagnosed on the basis of the pathogenic DNA. In a comparable manner, leishmaniasis can be identified and also typed by PCR and subsequent analysis of the amplified length of DNA can indicate the subspecies. *Borrelia burgdorferi*, the causative spirochaete of Lyme disease and erythema chronicum migrans, is present in very low amounts in infected tissue, but PCR may enable its detection as an alternative to diagnosis by seropositivity. Detection of antibodies is the usual method of the diagnosis of infection with RNA viruses, but again specific RT PCR of blood or tissue can allow earlier diagnosis.

CANCER

Diagnosis of skin cancers is achieved predominantly by the recognition of a combination of clinical and histopathological features, whilst their treatment depends largely on destruction by surgical excision or radiotherapy, or measures such as chemotherapy which rely for their effect on the higher proliferative rate of tumour cells. Even though these approaches are efficacious in many cases, certain skin cancers have a high mortality. The ability to identify individuals at risk of developing particular malignancies could permit focused screening and recognition of premalignant changes at an early stage. In cases of diagnostic uncertainty, clearer definition would lead to prompt but appropriate action and a better understanding of the steps of carcinogenesis would lead to the development of further therapeutic possibilities, hopefully with more specific action. Molecular medicine holds the key to at least some of these deficiencies.

Predisposition to some cancers is inherited. In the case of skin cancers, examples of familial syndromes include dysplastic naevi with malignant melanomas, the Li–Fraumeni syndrome and Gorlin's syndrome. The techniques of genetic linkage have shown that the most likely candidate gene for the predisposition to melanomas and dysplastic naevi lies on chromosome 9q, termed the MLM2 gene, with a less strong association with an area on chromosome 1, MLM 1. The hunt for the actual gene is now gradually focusing on more precise areas. The p53 gene, which has a role in control of cell cycling, has been identified as the site for mutations in the Li-Fraumeni syndrome, in which breast cancers, sarcomas and skin cancers are common. Gorlin's syndrome is an autosomal dominant condition in which skeletal abnormalities are found in association with skin changes of palmar pits and numerous basal cell carcinomas (BCCs) from an early age. Study of RFLPs in affected families has led to the identification of the site of the gene responsible for this syndrome. More recently, the nature of the gene product functionally lost in tumours of Gorlin's syndrone has been identified as a protein important in inhibiting expression of certain genes.

Many steps may be involved in the progression of a cell towards frank malignancy. Chromosomal changes have long been used as markers for certain tumours, e.g. the Philadelphia chromosome in which there is a translocation between chromosomes 9 and 22 in chronic myeloid leukaemia. Solid tumours may also exhibit chromosomal changes, but difficulties may be encountered in obtaining enough tissue for traditional chromosomal spreads. The use of PCR coupled with microsatellite markers has facilitated chromosomal analysis of very small pieces of tissue, including archival tissue which has been formalin-fixed and paraffin-embedded.

Diagnostic uncertainty can surround certain skin lesions, leading potentially to delay in appropriate treatment or inappropriate overtreatment. In lymphocytic infiltrates of the skin, the histological similarities between the benign infiltrates of Jessner's and lymphocytoma cutis and the malignant mycosis fungoides MF, cutaneous T-cell lymphoma may make precise diagnosis and prognosis difficult. Immunohistochemistry with lymphocyte markers can indicate the predominant cell type in the infiltrate but an indication of monoclonality can only be obtained by molecular analysis. The focus for this is the T-cell receptor gene, which shows great diversity in keeping with the vast array of lymphocytes produced to combat infections. In malignant cutaneous T-cell lymphomas, the infiltrating lymphocytes are monoclonal, in contrast to the polyclonal infiltrate in the benign diseases, with the exception of the monoclonal infiltrate of lymphomatoid papulosis, in which only about 10% of patients will develop MF. Southern blot hybridization of DNA extracted from biopsy samples can be used to determine monoclonality and, more recently, PCR amplification of specific portions of a variable region of part of the T-cell receptor gene can be used as an alternative.

INFLAMMATION

Cytokines, along with other putative mediators of inflammation, are believed to play an important role in inflammatory skin diseases, including psoriasis and atopic dermatitis. Molecular biology techniques have been useful in demonstrating that not only are certain cytokines present in lesional tissue, but that they are also likely to be synthesized *in situ*.

For example, interleukin-8 (IL-8) is present in scales from psoriatic lesions but not in uninvolved psoriatic or normal skin. High levels of IL-8 mRNA are found in psoriatic lesions using *in situ* hybridization, suggesting that keratinocytes in psoriatic tissue can synthesize IL-8. Protein kinase C inhibitors have been found to inhibit phorbol ester–stimulated IL-8 production in human keratinocytes *in vitro* and Northern analysis has shown inhibition of IL-8 mRNA.

Peripheral blood mononuclear leukocytes from patients with atopic dermatitis express higher levels of IL-4 receptor (IL-4R) mRNA and produce significantly higher amounts of T-cell-derived IL-4 than normal controls. Overstimulation of the IL-4–IL-4R pathway *in vivo* may account for

increased immunoglobulin E production in atopic diseases and this mechanism can be influenced therapeutically by administration of interferon-gamma. In addition, dermal eosinophils from lesional atopic dermatitis skin express IL-5 mRNA.

Measurement of cytokine secretion profiles can also allow the identification of pathogenetically important T cells in a particular disease. Using a PCR technique, psoriatic epidermal specimens have been shown to possess mRNA for the Th 1 cytokine interferon-gamma, but not for the Th 2 cytokines IL-4 and IL-10. This finding is not specific to psoriasis, however, since the neoplastic disease MF exhibits a Th 1-type cytokine profile, in this respect differing from the systemic T-cell disease Sézary syndrome, which expresses a Th 2 pattern.

THE FUTURE

How will molecular biology help in the practice of dermatology in the future? At present, many techniques remain as research tools rather than in mainstream laboratory diagnostics. The main impact is probably in the production of specifically targeted antibodies for use in immunocytochemistry and immunohistology. *In situ* hybridization is also becoming widespread, with the development of simple-to-use kits for rapid analysis. These have initially been rather expensive, but as prices come down their use in diagnostic laboratories will increase.

As research identifies the mechanisms underlying diseases, the possibility for greater precision of therapy increases. Iatrogenic immunosuppression is widely used to treat a vast array of immunologically mediated disease, but already attempts are being made to focus immunosuppression towards the specific lymphocytes mediating individual diseases. Antilymphocyte antibodies have been engineered against different forms of lymphocytes (identified by molecules expressed on their cell surface) and have been used therapeutically in psoriasis and cutaneous T-cell lymphoma.

If a specific gene (or genes) responsible for an

abnormality can be identified as being overactive, underactive or mutated, then the possibility for targeting that gene for therapy starts to become a possibility. Overactive genes or mutated genes producing the wrong product could be neutralized by the use of inhibitors of the promoter or by antisense oligonucleotides to block transcription from the mRNA. The proteins from underactive genes or absent genes could be replaced by expression in transfected DNA. At present one of the main drawbacks of gene therapy is the diffi-culty of delivering the genetic material into the required cells, ideally in a system which will keep it there. Several viruses, often in an attenuated form, have been tried as vectors for therapeutic genes, but there remains a risk of reversion to pathogenic variety. Some pilot studies of gene therapy in malignant melanoma are already underway. The future will no doubt bring many further attempts at gene therapy and refinement of techniques but it may take many years until such treatment becomes routine.

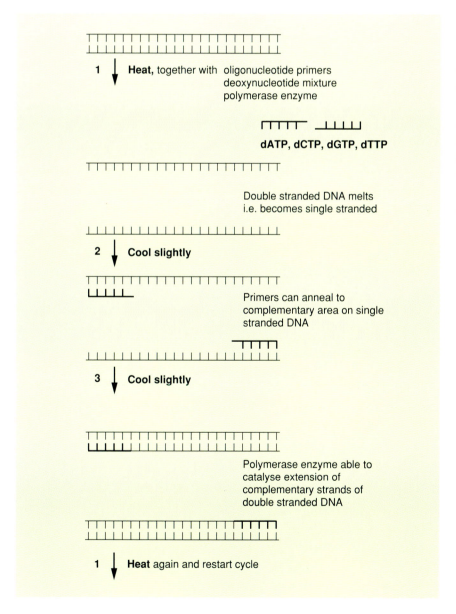

Fig. 10.9 Polymerase chain reaction. The template DNA is denatured by heat, but as it cools the available primers anneal to the complementary sequence. With a further reduction in temperature, the polymerase enzyme becomes active and can catalyse the chain extension reaction. When the temperature rises again, the newly made double-stranded DNA melts into single strands which in turn can undergo the same series of changes.

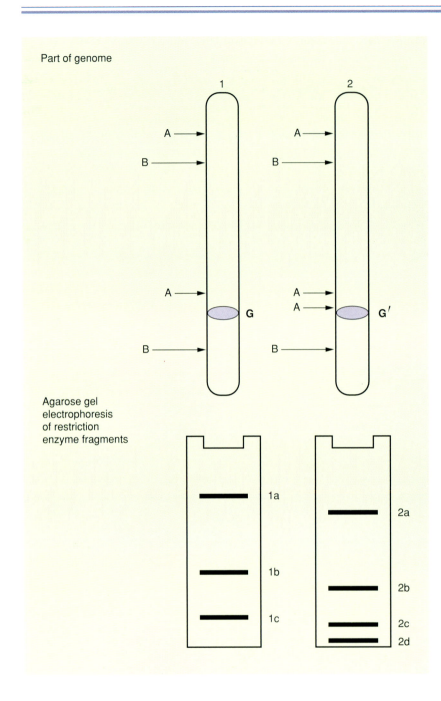

Part of genome

Agarose gel electrophoresis of restriction enzyme fragments

Fig. 10.10 Linkage analysis. In a search for a gene responsible for a particular disorder, a series of restriction enzyme digestions are analysed for a pattern of variation which is linked to the disease. In this scheme, the unknown gene is G. It is normal (G) in the chromosome of individual 1, but abnormal (G') in 2. Digestion of the DNA of individual 1 with restriction enzyme A produces three fragments, 1a, 1b and 1c. Due to a genetic variation adjacent to gene G in individual 2 there is one more site which the enzyme can cut and so four fragments 2a, 2b, 2c and 2d result. Fragments 1a and 1c are identical with fragments 2a and 2c. Restriction enzyme B produces the same fragment pattern in both individuals. As gene G' is very close to the site at which there is an extra cutting site for enzyme A, these two areas will be likely to be inherited together, whilst gene G will consistently be inherited with the length of genome with no additional cut site. If other affected individuals show the same pattern as B and unaffected individuals pattern A, then a **p**olymorphism of a **f**ragment **l**ength produced by a **r**estriction enzyme will have been demonstrated – RFLP – and the search for the gene can focus on the areas adjacent to the extra enzyme-cutting site.

FURTHER READING

Alberts B, Bray D, Lewis J, Raff M, Roberts K and Watson JD. *Molecular Biology of the Cell*, 2nd edn. Garland, New York, 1989.

Bahler D, Berry G, Okensberg J, Warnke R and Levy R. Diversity of T-cell antigen receptor variable genes used in mycosis fungoides cells. *American Journal of Pathology* 1992; **140**:1–8.

Chabot-Fletcher M, Breton J, Lee J, Young P and Griswold DE. Interleukin-8 production is regulated by protein kinase C in human keratinocytes. *Journal of Investigative Dermatology* 1994; **103**:509–515.

Fuchs E, Chan Y, Paller AS and Yu Q-C. Cracks in the foundation: keratin filaments and genetic disease. *Trends in Cell Biology* 1994; **4**:321–326.

Knox SJ, Levy R, Hodgkinson S *et al.* Observations

on the effect of chimeric anti-CD4 monoclonal antibody in patients with mycosis fungoides. *Blood* 1991; **77**:20–30.

Naber SP. Molecular pathology – diagnosis of infectious disease. *New England Journal of Medicine* 1994; **331**:1212–1215.

Raskø L and Downes CS. *Genes in Medicine. Molecular Biology and Human Genetic Disorders.* Chapman & Hall, London, 1995.

Renz H, Jujo K, Bradley KL, Domenico J, Gelfand EW and Leung DYM. Enhanced IL-4 production and IL-4 receptor expression in atopic dermatitis and their modulation by interferon-gamma. *Journal of Investigative Dermatology* 1992; **99**:403–408.

Saed G, Fivenson DP, Naidu Y and Nickoloff BJ. Mycosis fungoides exhibits a Th 1-type cell mediated cytokine profile whereas Sézary syndrome expresses a Th 2-type profile. *Journal of Investigative Dermatology* 1994; **103**:29–33.

Schlaak JF, Buslau MM, Jochum W *et al.* T cells involved in psoriasis vulgaris belong to the Th 1 subset. *Journal of Investigative Dermatology* 1994; **102**:145–149.

Schluger N, Kinney D, Harkin T, Rom W. Clinical utility of the polymerase chain reaction in the diagnosis of infections due to *Mycobacterium tuberculosis. Chest* 1994; **105**:1116–1121.

Sikora K. Genes, dreams and cancer. *British Medical Journal* 1994; **308**:1217–1221.

Index